Cambridge Clinical Guides

Hypertension in Pregnancy

Hypertension in Pregnancy

Edited by

Alexander Heazell
University of Manchester

Errol R. Norwitz
Yale University School of Medicine

Louise C. Kenny
University College Cork

Philip N. Baker
University of Alberta

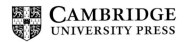

CAMBRIDGE UNIVERSITY PRESS
Cambridge, New York, Melbourne, Madrid, Cape Town, Singapore,
São Paulo, Delhi, Dubai, Tokyo, Mexico City

Cambridge University Press
The Edinburgh Building, Cambridge CB2 8RU, UK

Published in the United States of America by
Cambridge University Press, New York

www.cambridge.org
Information on this title: www.cambridge.org/9780521731560

First published 2010

Printed in the United Kingdom at the University Press, Cambridge

A catalog record for this publication is available from the British Library

Library of Congress Cataloging-in-Publication data

Hypertension in pregnancy / edited by Alexander Heazell ... [et al.].
   p. ; cm.
  Includes bibliographical references and index.
  ISBN 978-0-521-73156-0 (pbk.)
1. Hypertension in pregnancy. I. Heazell, Alexander. II. Title.
  [DNLM: 1. Hypertension. 2. Pregnancy Complications, Cardiovascular. 3. Pregnancy.
WQ 244 H9977 2010]
   RG580.H9H945 2010
   618.3′6132–dc22

                                          2010015187

ISBN 978-0-521-73156-0 Paperback

Contents

Color plate section between pp. 78 and 79.

Contributors

Philip N. Baker DM FRCOG
Faculty of Medicine & Dentistry
University of Alberta, Canada.

John Clift MBBS FRCA
City Hospital
Sandwell and West Birmingham NHS Trust
Birmingham, UK.

Ian Crocker PhD
Maternal and Fetal Health Research Centre
University of Manchester
St Mary's Hospital
Manchester, UK.

Edmund F. Funai MD
Dept of Obstetrics, Gynecology & Reproductive Sciences
Yale-New Haven Hospital
New Haven, CT, USA.

Alexander Heazell MBChB(Hons) PhD MRCOG
Maternal and Fetal Health Research Centre
University of Manchester
St Mary's Hospital
Manchester, UK.

Arun Jeyabalan MD
Magee-Womens Hospital
Pittsburgh, PA, USA.

S. Ananth Karumanchi, MD
Beth Israel Deaconess Medical Center
Boston, MA, USA.

Louise C. Kenny PhD MRCOG
Department of Obstetrics and Gynaecology
University College Cork
Cork, Ireland.

Mark Kilby MD FRCOG
School of Clinical & Experimental Medicine
University of Birmingham
Edgbaston
Birmingham, UK.

Ellen Knox MD MRCOG
Department of Fetal Medicine
Birmingham Women's Foundation Trust
Edgbaston
Birmingham, UK.

Fergus P. McCarthy MRCPI
Anu Research Centre
Cork University Maternity Hospital
Wilton
Cork, Ireland.

Fiona Milne
Action on Preeclampsia, PRECOG co-ordinator
Syston, UK.

Errol R. Norwitz MD PhD
Dept of Obstetrics, Gynecology & Reproductive Sciences
Yale-New Haven Hospital
New Haven, CT, USA.

Sarosh Rana MD
Division of Maternal-Fetal Medicine and Department
of Obstetrics and Gynecology
Beth Israel Deaconess Medical Center
Boston, MA, USA.

John T. Repke MD FACOG
Milton S. Hershey Medical Center
Hershey, PA, USA.

Baha M. Sibai, MD
Department of Obstetrics and Gynecology
University of Cincinnati
Cincinnati, OH, USA.

Stephen Thung
Yale University School of Medicine
New Haven, CT, USA.

Foreword

The management of hypertension during pregnancy presents a formidable challenge for the team managing the care of the pregnant woman and her infant. The editors of *Hypertension in Pregnancy* provide an excellent framework with which to meet this challenge. They bring to the subject a wealth of experience. I have observed the excellent work of Professors Baker, Kenny, and Norwitz for more than a decade. However, they have wisely included a new face, Dr Alex Heazell, one of the bright new clinician scientists in the area, for a fresh perspective. The editors have assembled an impressive group of experts from around the world to provide a practical guide to management that is nonetheless directed by state-of-the-art knowledge of pathophysiology. Having worked in this area for over 30 years I appreciate the importance as well as the difficulty of such an approach. The editors have included chapters addressing the normal physiology of pregnancy and the pathophysiology of hypertensive disorders to set the stage for the remainder of the book, which presents logical, evidence-based approaches to management. The team caring for the hypertensive mother and her fetus includes obstetricians, obstetrical physicians, anesthetists, and midwives. This information is crucial for the entire team and is presented in clearly written text with figures and tables making it useful to all.

In addition to the obviously important topics of acute management of all forms of pregnancy hypertension from several perspectives, the editors and authors address areas of increasing importance. These include exciting new information on screening and risk stratification. The editors have enlisted the leading experts in the discovery and development of screening strategies to address this topic. The presentation also addresses the very important topic of later-life implications of hypertensive disorders of pregnancy. All too frequently, individuals caring for women with pregnancy hypertension (myself included), after they have appropriately breathed a sigh of relief with a successful pregnancy outcome for the hypertensive mother and her offspring, do not appreciate that the implications of these disorders extend beyond pregnancy. Knowledge about later-life implications of all forms of preeclampsia has grown dramatically and this information is presented by the individuals responsible for these new insights. For example, the classic work of Leon Chesley suggesting that women who had eclampsia (and by extension well-characterized preeclampsia) in their first pregnancy did not have an increased risk for later-life cardiovascular disease has been modified to indicate increased risk for even these women by the excellent work of the authors of Chapter 12 regarding later-life implications of preeclampsia.

The bulk of the book, however, although guided by physiology and pathophysiology, is a practical "how to" presentation with chapters relating to the management of very specific issues. For example, separate chapters describe the management of severe and mild preeclampsia and also primary and secondary chronic hypertension.

The net result is a succinct but comprehensive set of evidence-based guidelines on the management of hypertension in pregnancy that should be on the reference shelves of all members of the team caring for women with these challenging conditions.

Professor Jim Roberts

Preface

Hypertension in pregnancy is an important topic which merits a focussed text. Hypertensive disorders of pregnancy are associated with increased maternal and perinatal morbidity and mortality, some of which may be preventable by appropriate clinical management. Care of women with hypertension in pregnancy, particularly those with preeclampsia, requires multidisciplinary management, including input from obstetricians, physicians, anesthesiologists, and midwives.

Good understanding and communication is vital to ensure clear, early decision making in clinical practice. This book aims to provide a solid background understanding of the physiological changes of normal pregnancy and the pathogenesis of preeclampsia. Building on this appreciation of normal and abnormal physiology, the management of gestational hypertension, preeclampsia, and eclampsia are discussed. Algorithms are included to provide evidence-based pathways for care. This text has been drawn together from leading clinicians and researchers from Europe and North America to provide up-to-date information for care-providers around the world. We are keen to receive comments or suggestions about the book. Feedback regarding omissions or developments in practice is crucial to the development of the book. If you have useful information, or better approaches please email us at hypertensioninpregnancy@gmail.com.

Alexander Heazell
Errol R. Norwitz
Louise C. Kenny
Philip N. Baker

Abbreviations

ACE	Angiotensin converting enzyme
ACTH	Adrenocorticotropic hormone
ADH	Antidiuretic hormone
ADMA	Asymmetric dimethylarginine
AFI	Amniotic fluid index
AFP	Alpha-fetoprotein
ALT	Alanine transaminase
ANP	Atrial naturetic peptide
APA	Aldosterone-producing adenoma
APTTR	Activated partial thromboplastin time
ARB	Angiotensin II receptor blocker
ARF	Acute renal failure
AST	Aspartate transaminase
AT1-AA	Angiotensin II receptor 1 autoantibodies
BMI	Body mass index
BP	Blood pressure
BPP	Biophysical profile
cGMP	cyclic guanosine monophosphate
CI	Confidence interval
COX	Cyclooxygenase
CPAP	Continuous positive airway pressure
CRH	Corticotropin releasing hormone
CRP	C-reactive protein
CSE	Combined spinal-epidural
CT	Computed tomography
CTG	Cardiotocograph
CVD	Cardiovascular disease
CVP	Central venous pressure
DAU	Day assessment unit

DIC	Disseminated intravascular coagulopathy
ECG	Electrocardiogram
ESR	Erythrocyte sedimentation rate
ESRD	End-stage renal disease
ET	Endothelin
FBC	Full blood count
FFA	Free fatty acids
FGR	Fetal growth restriction
FH	Familial hyperaldosteronism
FMD	Fibromuscular dysplasia
GFR	Glomerular filtration rate
GH	Gestational hypertension
GTT	Glucose tolerance test
hCG	Human chorionic gonadotropin
HDU	High dependency unit
HELLP	Hemolysis, elevated liver enzymes and low platelets
hPL	Human placental lactogen
ICAM-1	Inter-cellular adhesion molecule-1
IGF-1	Insulin-like growth factor-1
IGFBP-3	Insulin-like growth factor-binding globulin 3
IHA	Idiopathic hyperaldosteronism
IL	Interleukin
INR	International normalized ratio
IPPV	Intermittent positive pressure ventilation
IUGR	Intrauterine growth restriction
IV	Intravenous
LDL	Low-density lipoproteins
LR	Likelihood ratio
MAP	Mean arterial pressure
MoM	Multiples of median
MR	Magnetic resonance
NO	Nitric oxide
NST	Non-stress test
OR	Odds ratio
PAI	Plasminogen activator inhibitor
PAF	Platelet activating factor
PAPP-A	Pregnancy-associated plasma protein-A

PCEA	Patient controlled epidural analgesia
PCR	Protein:creatinine ratio
PCWP	Pulmonary capillary wedge pressure
PE	Preeclampsia
PET	Positron emission tomography
PGI_2	Prostacyclin
PI	Pulsatility index
PIH	Pregnancy-induced hypertension
PlGF	Placental growth factor
PP-13	Placental protein-13
PRECOG	Preeclampsia community guideline
RBF	Renal blood flow
RR	Risk ratio
RRT	Renal replacement therapy
sFlt-1	Soluble fms-like tyrosine kinase-1
sEng	Soluble endoglin
SGA	Small for gestational age
SPECT	Single photon emission CT
T4	Thyroxine
TG	Triglycerides
TGF	Transforming growth factor
TNFα	Tumor necrosis factor-alpha
t-PA	Tissue plasminogen activator
TPA-Ag	Tissue plasminogen activator antigen
T_3	Triodothyronine
VCAM-1	Vascular cell adhesion molecule-1
VEGF	Vascular endothelial growth factor
vWF	von Willebrand factor

Adaptations of maternal cardiovascular and renal physiology to pregnancy

Fergus P. McCarthy and Louise C. Kenny

■ Introduction

Major cardiovascular and renal changes occur during pregnancy to ensure optimal development of the placenta and fetus, and to protect the health of the mother. These changes include increases in the cardiac output and reductions in the systemic vascular resistance and systemic blood pressure. A clear understanding of all these changes is necessary in order to understand how disruptions in the normal physiological responses to pregnancy result in pathological conditions associated with pregnancy such as pregnancy-induced hypertension and preeclampsia.

■ Physiological hematological changes in pregnancy

To understand the cardiovascular changes which occur during pregnancy it is important to consider first of all the hematological changes that occur, as these will have an important influence on the changes which are required in pregnancy by the cardiovascular system.

Hypertension in Pregnancy, ed. Alexander Heazell, Errol R. Norwitz, Louise C. Kenny, and Philip N. Baker. Published by Cambridge University Press. © Cambridge University Press 2010.

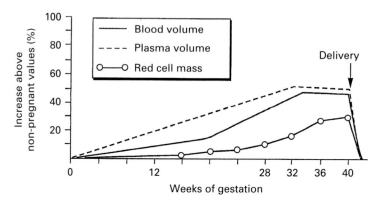

Figure 1.1 Increase in blood volume and its components in pregnancy.

Blood volume

In pregnancy, plasma volume increases by over a litre from 2600 mL to approximately 5000 mL. This occurs early in pregnancy and plateaus by approximately 32 weeks' gestation (Figure 1.1). This increase in plasma volume is approximate and correlates with the size of the fetus. Multiple pregnancies therefore are associated with a greater increase in plasma volume while pregnancies where the fetus is growth restricted are associated with a suboptimal increase in plasma volume. The blood volume in pregnant women at term is approximately 100 mL/kg [1].

Hematological indices

The red cell mass increases in a linear fashion by approximately 30% throughout pregnancy (Figure 1.1), from a non-pregnant level of 1400 mL to approximately 1700 mL [2]. The increase in cell mass is stimulated by increased erythropoietin synthesis and varies depending on the use of iron supplementation [3]. Plasma volume increases proportionately more than red cell mass and therefore the hematocrit and hemoglobin concentrations fall during pregnancy resulting in a physiological anemia. This physiological anemia becomes most apparent at 30–34 weeks when plasma volume peaks in relation to red cell volume. Although significant clinical effort is directed at reducing this physiological anemia, this and the hypervolemia that occurs in pregnancy are not without benefit. In fact, the absence of this physiological anemia is associated with a higher incidence of adverse pregnancy outcomes [4]. Physiological anemia and hypervolemia result in a decreased blood viscosity which in turn results in reduced resistance to flow therefore improving placenta perfusion and lowering cardiac workload. The term physiological anemia is misleading, as by the time the mother reaches full term, maternal blood volume has increased by approximately 50% above non-pregnant levels and the woman has a greater total hemoglobin than when non-pregnant to allow for any blood loss associated with delivery. Following delivery, placental separation, and uterine contractions approximately 500 mL of blood is transferred back to the maternal circulation from the uteroplacental unit to minimize any circulatory deficits which may result from blood loss at delivery. During pregnancy, iron is removed from the iron stores held in the bone marrow, the liver, and the spleen for use by the mother, and transferred to the fetus. This decrease in the quantity of stored iron is reflected in decreased serum ferritin levels.

In addition to changes in the red cell mass, there is also an increase in the white cell count and platelet count. The increase in white cell count is mainly due to an increase in neutrophil polymorphonuclear leukocytes and reaches its peak at 30 weeks' gestation. During labor there is a fourfold increase in the number of neutrophils but a fall in the number of eosinophils. During pregnancy lymphocyte function and cell-mediated immunity are profoundly suppressed resulting in a lowered resistance to viral infection.

The mean platelet count remains normal or decreases slightly in normal pregnancy, but platelet function does not appear to be altered. The serum protein pattern alters with total protein, albumin, and gamma globulin falling in the first quarter and then rising slowly towards term. Total protein concentration falls from approximately 70 g/L to 60 g/L with the decrease mainly due to a fall in albumin levels. Beta globulin and the fibrinogen factors rise causing a fourfold increase in the erythrocyte sedimentation rate (ESR) rendering this laboratory test difficult to interpret in pregnancy.

Coagulation factors

Pregnancy is a prothrombotic state and the majority of clotting factors either remain constant or increase during pregnancy. During the third trimester, plasma levels of von Willebrand factor are elevated promoting platelet aggregation and coagulation. Fibrinogen levels (factor I) increase significantly, in addition to factors II, V, VII, VIII, X, and XII. Protein S, an endogenous anticoagulant is reduced and there is an increase in the resistance to activated protein C. Endothelium production of the fibrinolytic inhibitors plasminogen activator inhibitor-1 (PAI-1) and PAI-2 increases, in addition to tissue plasminogen activator (t-PA). The net result of these changes are both inhibition and promotion of fibrinolysis respectively. Overall there is a 20% reduction in the prothrombin and the partial thromboplastin times.

■ Physiological cardiovascular changes in pregnancy

Cardiac output

An extra 30–50 mL of oxygen is consumed per minute during pregnancy and an increase in cardiac output is required to meet these extra demands. Stroke volume and heart rate are the two factors that govern cardiac output. The resting cardiac output in females is approximately 4.5 litres per minute. In pregnancy the cardiac output rises by approximately 40% to 6 litres per minute (Figure 1.2). This change occurs early in pregnancy with one half of this increase occurring prior to 8 weeks' gestation. The increase in cardiac output plateaus at 20–30 weeks' gestation. Heart rate increases during pregnancy from 80 beats per minute to 90 beats per minute further contributing to the required increase in cardiac output [5]. In addition there is a decrease in the arteriovenous oxygen gradient, an increase in the preload due to the increase in blood volume, and a reduction in the afterload due to the decline in systemic vascular resistance [6]. The increased cardiac output is distributed throughout the body with the uterus receiving approximately 400 mL/min extra and the kidneys receiving approximately 300 mL/min extra.

During labor significant hemodynamic changes occur due to anxiety, exertion, pain, uterine contractions, uterine involution, and bleeding. These changes may be more significant if the woman is exposed to infection, hemorrhage, or the administration of anesthesia or analgesia. During labor blood from the uterine sinusoids is forced into the systemic circulation with each uterine contraction, thereby increasing preload during labor. Cardiac output increases by 15% above pre-labor levels

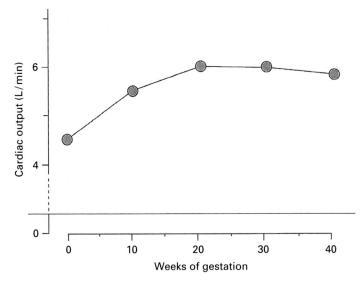

Figure 1.2 Cardiac output in pregnancy. The increase occurs very early and plateaus from approximately 20 weeks of pregnancy.

in early labor and by approximately 25% during the active phase. The additional exertion associated with pushing in the second stage results in a 50% rise in cardiac output. Immediately postpartum, cardiac output increases to 80% above pre-labor values due to significant auto-transfusion associated with uterine involution. It takes approximately three months for the cardiac output and systemic vascular resistance to return to non-pregnant levels.

Blood pressure regulation

In the absence of any pathological process such as preeclampsia, blood pressure remains relatively constant throughout pregnancy. Despite the increases observed in cardiac output, systolic and diastolic blood pressure may drop slightly by up to 5 mmHg and 10 mmHg respectively in the second trimester (Figure 1.3). This occurs due to a decrease in peripheral resistance which exceeds the increase in cardiac output. This decrease in total peripheral resistance accommodates the increased blood flow which is required by various organs and results from a generalized vasodilatation that occurs during pregnancy. The drop

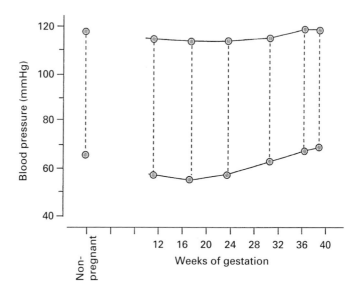

Figure 1.3 Systolic and diastolic blood pressures during pregnancy. The mid-trimester dip found in some women is seen more in the diastolic than in the systolic pressure.

in blood pressure observed in the second trimester recovers, and by term blood pressure levels have returned to normal pre-pregnancy ranges. Central venous pressures, pulmonary capillary wedge pressures, and pulmonary artery systolic and diastolic pressures all remain at a non-pregnant level as increases in cardiac preload and hypervolemia of pregnancy are counterbalanced by falls in both the pulmonary vascular resistance and systemic vascular resistance.

Peripheral resistance is controlled neurogenically by the autonomic nervous system, and directly by substances that act on the blood vessels. These include angiotensin II, serotonin, kinins, catecholamines secreted from the adrenal medulla, metabolites such as adenosine, potassium, hydrogen ions, prostaglandins, and changes in partial pressures of carbon dioxide and oxygen.

In labor and throughout the late second and third trimesters of pregnancy women are advised not to lie directly supine as the gravid uterus compresses the inferior vena cava and decreases the venous return decreasing the cardiac output resulting in hypotension (supine hypotensive syndrome). This hypotension may result in fetal distress secondary to reduced uteroplacental perfusion.

Role of the endothelium in the cardiovascular system

In normal pregnancy the endothelium undergoes many subtle changes in function which contribute to the maintenance of normal cardiovascular function in the mother. The maternal vascular endothelium has many important functions including control of smooth muscle tone through release of vasoconstrictor and vasodilatory substances and regulation of anticoagulation, antiplatelet, and fibrinolytic functions via the release of different soluble factors. The endothelium synthesizes a number of potent vasoactive factors which influence the tone of the underlying vascular smooth muscle. These vasoactive factors include the vasoconstrictors endothelin, angiotensin, and thromboxane. The vasodilators include agents such as nitric oxide (NO) and prostacyclin (PGI_2), the levels of which increase considerably in pregnancy.

In conditions such as preeclampsia there is an abnormal shift towards vasoconstriction. The clinical features of pathological conditions including preeclampsia can be explained as clinical responses to generalized endothelial dysfunction, e.g., hypertension results from disturbed endothelial control of vascular tone, while proteinuria and edema are caused by increased vascular permeability, and coagulopathy is the result of abnormal endothelial expression of procoagulants [7,8]. Underlying endothelial dysfunction is evidenced by decreases in the production of NO and PGI_2, increased production of endothelin, thrombomodulin, and thromboxane, and enhanced vascular reactivity to angiotensin II.

Thromboxane is a member of the eicosanoid family and is produced in platelets by thromboxane-A synthase from the endoperoxides produced by the cyclooxygenase (COX) enzyme from arachidonic acid. Thromboxane acts by binding to any of the thromboxane receptors, which are G protein-coupled receptors coupled to the G protein G_q. Thromboxane is a vasoconstrictor and a potent hypertensive agent, and facilitates platelet aggregation. It is in homeostatic balance in the circulatory system with PGI_2, a related compound. Significant alterations in PGI_2 and thromboxane production occur in women with preeclampsia with studies demonstrating a shift in the renal and vascular PGI_2/thromboxane A_2 ratio towards thromboxane A_2 production, resulting in a tendency to vasoconstriction. Decreases in plasma levels of PGI_2 in women with preeclampsia have been demonstrated as early as 13 weeks' gestation. Prostacyclin is the predominant vasodilator in pregnancy and is derived from the arachidonic acid pathway after conversion by COX.

The endothelin (ET) family consists of three 21-amino acid peptides (ET-1, ET-2, and ET-3). Endothelins are produced by most cell types in the kidney and have a wide variety of biological actions including regulation of vascular resistance, modulation of fluid and electrolyte transport, and regulation of cell proliferation and extracellular matrix accumulation. Endothelin-1 plays the predominant physiological role in the control of vascular tone and is a highly potent vasoconstrictor agonist. Endothelial damage is a known stimulus for ET-1 synthesis. It is speculated that increases in the production of ET-1 may be involved in the pathogenesis of preeclampsia. These elevated plasma levels of ET-1, which are two- to threefold increased in pregnancy-induced hypertension may have significant long-term effects on systemic hemodynamic and arterial pressure regulation.

Endothelium-derived NO is a key molecule in vascular biology since it is capable of reducing vascular tone, smooth muscle cell proliferation, leukocyte adhesion, and platelet aggregation. Nitric oxide causes relaxation in vascular smooth muscle through activation of soluble guanylate cyclase and subsequent stimulation of cyclic guanosine monophosphate (cGMP). Substantial evidence indicates that NO production is elevated in normal pregnancy and that these increases appear to play an important role in the renal vasodilatation of pregnancy [9]. The increase in NO may be mediated via the ovarian hormone and vasodilator relaxin. The plasma concentration of relaxin rises during pregnancy, a response mediated by human chorionic gonadotropin (hCG). Relaxin is a peptide hormone in the insulin family and it is normally produced in the corpus luteum, but in pregnancy is produced in large amounts by the placenta and decidua. Chronic administration of relaxin to conscious male and castrated female rats mimics the renal hemodynamic changes of pregnancy (20–40% increase in glomerular filtration rate [GFR] and renal plasma flow). These changes are abolished by the administration of a NO synthase inhibitor. The increases in GFR and renal plasma flow in pregnant rats can also be abolished by the administration of antirelaxin antibodies [10].

The actions of hormones derived from the adrenal gland and placenta also appear to play a role in the regulation of blood pressure in normal pregnancy. There is a significant increase in aldosterone levels by the eighth week of pregnancy and this continues to rise to 80 to 100 ng/dL in the third trimester, fourfold to sixfold above the upper limits observed in non-pregnant adults. Progesterone levels parallel those of aldosterone, reaching a level of 200 ng/dL by term. It is likely that aldosterone is critical in maintaining the sodium balance in the setting of vasodilatation of the peripheral vasculature.

■ Maternal renal physiological changes in pregnancy

Normal pregnancy is characterized by increased renal perfusion and several, usually minor changes in extracellular composition, including chronic respiratory alkalosis and hyponatremia [5]. Increased renal perfusion is attributable to the increased cardiac output that occurs during pregnancy.

Renal anatomy

The kidneys increase in size by approximately 1 cm in length secondary to an increase in renal vascular and interstitial volume as opposed to an increase in the number of nephrons. Ureteric dilatation occurs secondary to obstruction of the ureters by the gravid uterus and the smooth muscle relaxation which occurs due to increased circulating levels of progesterone [11]. These raised circulating levels of progesterone also decrease peristalsis and contraction pressure. This dilatation of the upper ureters and pelvic calyces is referred to as the physiological hydroureter of pregnancy. The hydronephrosis which occurs in pregnancy occurs predominantly on the right-hand side (90% vs. 10%). This preference of the right side is most likely explained by anatomical factors. These include dextrorotation of the uterus by the sigmoid colon, kinking of the ureter as it crosses the right iliac artery, and the proximity of the ureter to the right ovarian vein. In addition to the dilatation of the proximal ureters there may also be distal dilatation. The vessels in the suspensory ligament of the ovary enlarge and may compress the ureter at the brim of the bony pelvis, thus causing dilatation above that level. Hypertrophy of Waldeyer's sheath (i.e., the longitudinal muscle bundles in the lower ureter) causes mild stenosis in the juxtavesical region, thereby contributing to dilatation of the ureter above the pelvic brim. These changes result in a physiological dilated collecting system which leads to an accumulation of 200–300 mL of urine in the collecting system, and this urinary stasis in addition to an increased incidence of vesicoureteric reflux explains why the incidence of urinary tract infections and pyelonephritis increases in pregnancy. The physiological dilatation that occurs also renders ultrasound examination of the renal tract difficult as the only way to differentiate pathological from physiological change is by visualizing the obstruction, which often is not possible with ultrasound alone. During pregnancy the bladder becomes an intra-abdominal organ. Bladder capacity is also decreased by the enlarging uterus which displaces the bladder superiorly and anteriorly.

Ascertainment of symptoms as a sole means of eliciting a urinary tract infection in pregnancy is inadequate as studies have shown that urinary symptoms such as dysuria, polyuria, nocturia, urgency, and stress incontinence occur more frequently during pregnancy even in the absence of pathology [12]. Urinary frequency and nocturia are the commonest urinary symptoms in pregnancy. The increase in urinary frequency most likely occurs due to a combination of increased total urinary output, raised total plasma volume, increases in renal blood flow (RBF) and GFR, and occasionally higher fluid intake [13]. The increased incidence of nocturia in pregnancy appears to result from increased excretion of sodium and solute during the night in pregnancy compared to that in non-pregnant women.

Renal physiology

Renal blood flow rises markedly during pregnancy. It increases by 75–80% above non-pregnant values to at least 1.5 L/min in pregnancy and this change is evident within the first trimester. Glomerular filtration rate rises from 140 to 170 mL/min and similar to the RBF the increase in GFR can be demonstrated within one month of conception and reaches a peak approximately 40–50% above baseline levels by the end of the first trimester [14]. The increase in GFR is due solely to an increase in glomerular plasma flow and not increased intraglomerular capillary pressure. With the increase in GFR, there is an increase in endogenous clearance of creatinine.

Antidiuretic hormone (ADH) activates the vasopressin-2 receptor on the renal collecting ducts to stimulate water absorption. The release of vasopressinases from the placenta results in an approximate fourfold increase rate of ADH catabolism. However, plasma levels of ADH remain normal because of a fourfold rise in the production of ADH by the pituitary gland. Most women can increase ADH release to maintain sufficient antidiuretic activity to prevent polyuria, which is rare during pregnancy. However, intense polyuria and polydipsia can occur or be exacerbated in women with overt or subclinical central or nephrogenic diabetes insipidus in whom secretory reserve or renal responsiveness is impaired. The rise in GFR during pregnancy also may play a contributory role.

Renal biochemistry

In pregnancy plasma osmolality falls to a new set point of approximately 270 mOsm/kg. The physiological response to changes in osmolality above or below this new set point is compatible with the non-pregnant state. As an example, the plasma sodium concentration falls by about 5 mEq/L during pregnancy, a response that represents downward resetting of the osmoreceptor system (osmostat) [15]. Despite this reduction in serum sodium concentration there is retention of approximately 1000 mEq of sodium in addition to 6–8 litres of water during pregnancy. The fall in the plasma sodium concentration during pregnancy correlates closely with increased release of hCG. These changes to plasma sodium concentrations spontaneously rise to pre-pregnancy levels within one to two months after delivery [15,16].

Plasma creatinine is reduced by approximately 25% (falls from 73 to 54 mol/L) in proportion to the increase in GFR, and concentration of plasma urea is similarly reduced (from 4.3 to 3.1 mmol/L). The creatinine clearance increases to approximately 120–160 mL/min in pregnancy. Plasma renin concentration, renin activity, and angiotensin II levels are elevated in normal pregnancy but the vascular sensitivity to their hypertensive effects appears reduced. In contrast to the rise in plasma renin, atrial natriuretic peptide levels are slightly reduced. Renin is a proteolytic enzyme synthesized by the juxtaglomerular apparatus of the kidney and the pregnant uterus, which acts on a substrate of α-2-globulin to produce angiotensin I. There is a two and a half fold increase in plasma renin concentration by the first 12 weeks of pregnancy. Under the action of angiotensin converting enzyme (ACE) produced predominantly in the lung but also by the placenta, angiotensin I is converted to angiotensin II, a potent vasoconstrictor which also stimulates the release of aldosterone.

Pregnancy also alters renal tubular function. The fractional absorption of glucose, amino acids, and beta microglobulin is decreased, which results in higher rates of urinary excretion.

Protein excretion

Total urinary protein excretion rises in normal pregnancy from the non-pregnant level of about 100 mg to about 180–200 mg per 24 hours in the third trimester. This may result in a "positive" dipstick, e.g., + when a concentrated urine sample is examined. However, a positive dipstick for protein should warrant further investigation either in the form of a mid-stream urine for culture and sensitivity to exclude a urinary tract infection or a 24-hour collection to help outrule the diagnosis of preeclampsia (24-hour urine collection < 300 mg/24 hours [17]).

■ Signs and symptoms of cardiovascular and renal physiological changes in pregnancy

Physicians should be aware of the many symptoms experienced by pregnant women that result from the normal physiological changes of pregnancy, and unless severe do not warrant further investigation.

Pregnant women are more likely to suffer from breathlessness, fatigue, decreased exercise tolerance, and peripheral edema while many of the effects of the altered cardiovascular system mimic heart failure (edema, dyspnoea, distended neck veins). Here we will present a spectrum of clinical changes that occur antenatally and in labor that are associated with the normal renal and physiological adaptations to pregnancy.

Hyperventilation

In pregnancy, hyperventilation occurs due to stimulation of the central respiratory centers by progesterone. In a non-pregnant state this hyperventilation would result in a respiratory alkalosis with a low partial pressure of carbon dioxide and a rise in the pH. However, in pregnancy, the kidney excretes sufficient bicarbonate to compensate fully for the fall in carbon dioxide levels and there is no overall change in pH.

"Hot flushes/sweat easily/nasal congestion"

The blood flow through the skin and mucous membranes also increases during pregnancy reaching a maximum of approximately 500 mL per minute by the 36th week of gestation. Early in pregnancy, uterine blood flow has not increased although cardiac output and RBF have. There is therefore a disproportionately higher quantity of extra blood perfusing skin, breasts, and other organs. This increased flow is associated with peripheral vasodilatation which manifests itself clinically as nasal congestion and "feeling hot and sweaty."

Edema

There is a high incidence of edema in normal pregnancies due to an increase in fluid transfer across the endothelium. This may be due to an increase in the balance of transcapillary hydrostatic pressure favoring outward fluid transduction, or from a combination of this and increased fluid conductivity.

Varicosities

As with other vessels in the body, the veins of the legs become more distensible and with the obstruction of the venous return by the mechanical obstruction of the gravid uterus and the higher pressure of blood returning from the uterine veins, the venous pressure rises and pregnant women are more likely to suffer from varicose veins.

Heart sounds

At the beginning of ventricular systole the mitral valve is open and the pressure in the left atrium is greater than that in the left ventricle. As ventricular systole continues, the pressure in the left ventricle exceeds that in the left atrium and the mitral valve closes generating the first heart sound. Following this the pressure in the left ventricle exceeds that in the aorta and this opens the aortic valve resulting in the ejection of blood from the left ventricle. The ventricle then starts to relax and the pressure within the left ventricle falls. This fall in pressure results in the aortic valve closing generating the second heart sound. A third heart sound is commonly heard in pregnancy and is not considered pathological. It is lower in pitch than the first and second heart sounds and is not valvular in origin. It occurs at the beginning of diastole and results from a period of rapid ventricular filling. Auscultatory changes accompanying normal gestation begin in the late first trimester and generally disappear within a week after delivery. Dilatation across the tricuspid valve may result in mild regurgitant flow causing a normal grade I or II systolic murmur. In addition there may be a higher basal heart rate, louder heart sounds, wide splitting of S1, and splitting of S2 in the third trimester.

Blood pressure

Blood pressure may be observed to rise in labor due to uterine contractions expelling blood from the uterus, increasing cardiac output resulting in an increase in blood pressure.

Supine hypotension syndrome

This is discussed earlier and may be avoided by never allowing a woman to lie directly supine during pregnancy. When managing a pregnant patient, placing a wedge under the woman's right side, having the patient lie on her left side, or adjusting the operating table to a 30° left lateral tilt results in displacement of the uterus to the left and off the inferior vena cava therefore preventing this hypotension [18].

Glycosuria

Some patients may exhibit glycosuria in the absence of hyperglycemia because the raised GFR increases the filtered load of glucose and the fractional absorption may be decreased, resulting in increased urinary glucose excretion. Persistent or heavy glycosuria should prompt the patient to have a glucose tolerance test to exclude gestational diabetes mellitus.

Renal function

Physicians should be aware of the alterations in plasma creatinine (falls from 73 to 54 μmol/L) and plasma urea (falls from 4.3 to 3.1 mmol/L) as levels which may be considered normal outside of pregnancy may indicate renal disease in pregnancy.

Jugular venous pulse and cardiac changes

The jugular venous pulse is more obvious later in pregnancy but the mean jugular venous pressure remains normal. Palpation of the heart is difficult, particularly in advanced pregnancy due to enlargement of the breasts and abdomen. In pregnancy the heart is shifted to the left and anteriorly as the uterus enlarges. As a result, the apical impulse is shifted from its normal location in the fourth or fifth intercostal space along the midclavicular line, upwards and outwards to the fourth intercostal space and lateral to the midclavicular line.

Electrocardiogram

The physiological and anatomical changes that occur in pregnancy result in changes on an electrocardiogram (ECG). The heart is enlarged by both chamber dilatation and hypertrophy. The changes in location of the apex beat result in common ECG findings of left axis deviation, sagging ST segments, and frequently inversion or flattening of the T-wave in lead III. Periods of supraventricular tachycardia and ventricular extrasystoles may also be identified but should not be regarded as pathological changes.

Chest X-ray

The rotation of the heart and hypervolemia which occur in pregnancy may suggest ventricular hypertrophy and cardiomegaly on chest X-ray. Occasionally on chest radiographs enlarged pulmonary vessels are seen due to venous dilatation also occurring in the pulmonary vasculature.

■ Conclusion

Significant cardiovascular and renal adaptations occur in pregnancy to allow the fetus to achieve optimal growth while maintaining the well-being of both the fetus and the mother. A good understanding of these physiological adaptations is essential to help the physician appropriately manage a woman throughout her pregnancy. Pathological conditions which occur in pregnancy manifest as disruptions to these normal sequences of events. For example, preeclampsia is associated with a rise in total peripheral resistance, reduced cardiac output, reduced uteroplacental blood flow, increased mean arterial pressure, enhanced responsiveness to angiotensin II, proteinuria, and reductions in renal blood flow and glomerular filtration rate.

Only by understanding these normal physiological changes will a physician be able to understand and manage these abnormal pathological processes which may occur in pregnancy.

REFERENCES

1. Jansen AJ, van Rhenen DJ, Steegers EA, Duvekot JJ. Postpartum hemorrhage and transfusion of blood and blood components. *Obstet Gynecol Surv* 2005;**60**(10):663–71.
2. Llewellyn-Jones D. *Fundamentals of Obstetrics and Gynaecology*, 5th edn. Vol. 1 Obstetrics. London, Faber and Faber, 1990.
3. Milman N, Graudal N, Nielsen OJ, Agger AO. Serum erythropoietin during normal pregnancy: relationship to hemoglobin and iron status markers and impact of iron supplementation in a longitudinal, placebo-controlled study on 118 women. *Int J Hematol* 1997;**66**(2):159–68.
4. Stephansson O, Dickman PW, Johansson A, Cnattingius S. Maternal hemoglobin concentration during pregnancy and risk of stillbirth. *JAMA* 2000;**284**(20):2611–17.
5. de Swiet M, Chamberlain G, Bennett P. (eds.), *Basic Science in Obstetrics and Gynaecology*, 3rd edn. London, Churchill Livingstone, 2002.
6. Robson SC, Hunter S, Boys RJ, Dunlop W. Serial study of factors influencing changes in cardiac output during human pregnancy. *Am J Physiol* 1989;**256**(4 Pt 2):H1060–5.
7. Redman CW, Sacks GP, Sargent IL. Preeclampsia: an excessive maternal inflammatory response to pregnancy. *Am J Obstet Gynecol* 1999;**180**(2 Pt 1): 499–506.
8. Roberts JM, Taylor RN, Musci TJ, *et al.* Preeclampsia: an endothelial cell disorder. *Am J Obstet Gynecol* 1989;**161**(5):1200–4.
9. Sladek SM, Magness RR, Conrad KP. Nitric oxide and pregnancy. *Am J Physiol* 1997;**272**(2 Pt 2):R441–63.
10. Novak J, Danielson LA, Kerchner LJ, *et al.* Relaxin is essential for renal vasodilation during pregnancy in conscious rats. *J Clin Invest* 2001;**107**(11):1469–75.
11. Beydoun SN. Morphologic changes in the renal tract in pregnancy. *Clin Obstet Gynecol* 1985;**28**(2):249–56.
12. Nel JT, Diedericks A, Joubert G, Arndt K. A prospective clinical and urodynamic study of bladder function during and after pregnancy. *Int Urogynecol J Pelvic Floor Dysfunct* 2001;**12**(1):21–6.
13. Thorp JM, Jr., Norton PA, Wall LL, *et al.* Urinary incontinence in pregnancy and the puerperium: a prospective study. *Am J Obstet Gynecol* 1999;**181**(2): 266–73.

14. Davison JM, Dunlop W. Renal hemodynamics and tubular function normal human pregnancy. *Kidney Int* 1980;**18**(2):152–61.

15. Lindheimer MD, Barron WM, Davison JM. Osmoregulation of thirst and vaso-pressin release in pregnancy. *Am J Physiol* 1989;**257**(2 Pt 2):F159–69.

16. Lindheimer MD, Barron WM, Davison JM. Osmotic and volume control of vasopressin release in pregnancy. *Am J Kidney Dis* 1991;**17**(2):105–11.

17. Roberts JM, Pearson GD, Cutler JA, Lindheimer MD. National Heart Lung and Blood Institute. Summary of the NHLBI Working Group on Research on Hypertension During Pregnancy. *Hypertens Pregnancy* 2003;**22**(2):109–27.

18. Kinsella SM, Lohmann G. Supine hypotensive syndrome. *Obstet Gynecol* 1994;**83**(5 Pt 1):774–88.

The pathophysiology of hypertension in pregnancy

2

Ian Crocker and Alexander Heazell

■ The pathophysiology of hypertension

There remains much uncertainty about the pathophysiology of hypertension. A small number of patients (between 2% and 5%) have underlying renal or adrenal disease as the cause for their raised blood pressure. In the remainder, no clear single cause is identified and their condition is labeled "essential hypertension." A number of physiological mechanisms are involved in the maintenance of normal blood pressure, and their derangement may play a role in the development of essential hypertension.

It is likely that a great many interrelated factors will contribute to raised blood pressure in hypertensive patients, and their relative roles may differ between individuals. Among the factors intensively studied are salt intake, insulin resistance and obesity, the renin–angiotensin system, and the sympathetic nervous system. More recently other factors have been evaluated, including genetics, endothelial dysfunction, neurovascular anomalies, low birthweight, and insufficient intrauterine nutrition – the so called "Barker hypothesis" [1].

Patients with hypertension demonstrate abnormalities of their vessel walls (endothelial dysfunction or damage), blood constituents (abnormal levels of hemostatic factors, platelet activation, and fibrinolysis), and blood flow (rheology, viscosity, and flow reserve), suggesting that hypertension confers a prothrombotic or hypercoagulatory state. These components appear to be related to target organ damage and long-term

Hypertension in Pregnancy, ed. Alexander Heazell, Errol R. Norwitz, Louise C. Kenny, and Philip N. Baker. Published by Cambridge University Press. © Cambridge University Press 2010.

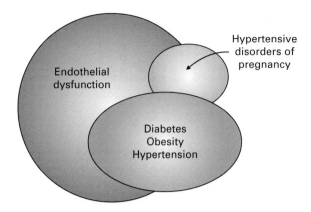

Figure 2.1 Endothelial dysfunction is common to both vascular complications and several hypertensive disorders of pregnancy, particularly preeclampsia. Metabolic and physiological changes in pregnancy may unmask underlying endothelial dysfunction, leading to the clinical syndrome of preeclampsia. Preeclamptic patients are also at a higher risk of developing vascular disease in later life.

prognosis, and some, but certainly not all, may be altered by antihypertensive treatment.

Epidemiologically there is a clustering of several risk factors, including obesity, glucose intolerance, diabetes mellitus, and hyperlipidemia, and this has led to the suggestion that these represent a single metabolic syndrome, with a final common pathway to raised blood pressure and vascular damage (see Figure 2.1). Indeed some hypertensive patients who are not obese still display resistance to insulin. Although there are many objections to this hypothesis, this may help explain why the hazards of cardiovascular risk are synergistic or multiplicative rather than just additive.

■ The vascular stress test of pregnancy

The maternal cardiovascular system undergoes a series of important physiological changes in pregnancy, most notably a significant increase in plasma volume (approximately 2600 to 3800 ml by 32 weeks' gestation) and cardiac output from increased stroke volume (4.5 L/min to 6 L/min by 30 weeks' gestation). Despite this increase, blood pressure falls until around 20 weeks' gestation before rising slowly towards term. This fall reflects a substantial reduction in total peripheral resistance, which counteracts cardiac output and enhances blood flow to the uterus and kidneys.

In addition to these adaptations, a pregnant woman experiences an increase in hypercoagulability and inflammatory activity and a degree of insulin resistance and dyslipidemia, again after 20 weeks' gestation. These adaptations serve to meet the metabolic needs of the growing fetus. It is noteworthy that all of these features are more pronounced in women with pregnancy-induced hypertension and preeclampsia.

Healthy pregnancy therefore transiently propels a woman into a metabolic syndrome that predisposes her to vascular endothelial dysfunction. Women already prone to this phenotype develop gestational hypertension or diabetes mellitus, which may reemerge in subsequent pregnancies or later life. Indeed, women who succumb to preeclampsia or pregnancy-induced hypertension are subsequently at increased risk of developing cardiovascular disease in adulthood [2]. The vascular stress test of pregnancy therefore identifies women with an unrecognized risk of vascular complications and these typical adaptive responses are exaggerated in preeclampsia, leading to more gross metabolic disturbances.

■ Common features of the metabolic syndrome of preeclampsia

There are generally considered to be five metabolic and systemic alterations involved in the pathophysiology of preeclampsia, namely endothelial dysfunction and activation, a systemic inflammatory response, oxidative stress, insulin resistance, and dyslipidemia. It is likely that these factors are not completely independent but rather interact in a patient-specific way. This in part, explains the enigmatic nature of the syndrome and difficulties in identifying mechanistic links.

Endothelial dysfunction and activation

The maternal vascular endothelium, the single-cell lining that covers the luminal side of blood vessels, is the dominant pathogenic target in preeclampsia, resulting in high blood pressure and glomerular endotheliosis, the classic renal lesion of the condition. The strategic location of the endothelium permits an active response to signal alterations in hemodynamics and humoral factors by synthesizing and releasing vaso-regulatory substances. Thus a critical balance between endothelium-derived relaxing and contracting factors maintains vascular homeostasis. When this balance is disrupted (as in preeclampsia) the vasculature becomes predisposed to irregular constriction and additionally leukocyte adherence, mitogenesis, pro-oxidation, and vascular inflammation.

In the non-pregnant state, vascular endothelial cells release vasodilators, such as nitric oxide (NO) and prostacyclin (PGI$_2$), and vasoconstrictors, such as endothelin (ET) and platelet activating factor (PAF), to regulate blood flow and pressure. Normal pregnancy is associated with reduced vascular reactivity and tone and therefore a predominance of vasodilatation. The in vivo and ex vivo assessment of endothelial-dependent vascular function in women with preeclampsia shows an opposite reaction to vasodilatory agents, more typical of the non-pregnant response [3,4]. Importantly, this endothelial dysfunction develops before the clinical onset of disease.

Circulating markers indicative of endothelial disruption in preeclampsia include plasminogen activator inhibitor-1 (PAI-1), von Willebrand factor (vWF), a range of cytokines, and soluble adhesion molecules (vascular cell adhesion molecule-1 [VCAM-1], inter-cellular adhesion molecule-1 [ICAM-1], and E-selectin). Likewise, circulating ET is reportedly elevated, suggestive of endothelial activation, along with thromboxane and superoxide anions, both vasoconstrictors [5]. An increase in endothelial sensitivity to constrictor agents, such as angiotensin II has also been reported, along with decreased formation of vasodilators, NO and PGI$_2$. Nevertheless, many of these findings and markers remain controversial.

Systemic inflammation and coagulation

Normal uncomplicated pregnancy is associated with a generalized maternal inflammatory response [6]. The maternal white cell count is elevated across gestation, attributed largely to neutrophilia, and there is generalized activation of neutrophils and other circulating leukocytes. Plasma cytokine levels (such tumor necrosis factor-alpha [TNFα], interleukin [IL]-2, IL-6, and IL-8) are elevated along with intracellular adhesion molecules, such as ICAM-1 and VCAM-1, and other acute phase inflammatory markers, such as C-reactive protein (CRP). This proposes an exaggerated inflammatory response in preeclampsia, much akin to sepsis, which is evident before clinical onset and diagnosis [7].

Neutrophil activation has been implicated in the pathophysiology of preeclampsia, for which several potential mechanisms have been defined, including TNFα activation, the upregulation of endothelial cell adhesion molecules (selectins and intergrins), and a direct response to circulating placental fragments (see further discussions below). Neutrophils are considered to contribute to maternal vascular dysfunction by releasing damaging enzymes and toxic oxygen radicals, which can encourage lipid peroxidation, lysis of endothelial cells, and increased vascular permeability and reactivity.

In addition to promoting endothelial damage, neutrophils interact with platelets and the coagulation and complement systems, all elements integral to the preeclamptic pathology. In normal pregnancy there are increases in coagulatory factors V, VII, VIII, vWF, X, and XII, an increase in plasma fibrinogen, and suppression of fibrinolysis, presumably to limit life-threatening bleeding at delivery [8]. In preeclampsia, VII activity and vWF are further increased and activation of the coagulation system which occurs often antedates clinical symptoms and is consistent with increased fibrin deposition and microvascular thrombi in many organs. Platelet activation, defined in the condition, may promote vascular obstruction, tissue ischemia, and further endothelial malfunction. Moreover, an additional depletion in circulating platelets is believed to reflect a reduction in platelet lifespan, whilst a concomitant increase in platelet-specific B thromboglobulin, a marker for platelet activation, has been correlated with proteinuria and is suggestive of platelet hyperactivation [9].

Oxidative stress

The oxidative stress theory of preeclampsia proposes that abnormal placentation and dyslipidemia results in the release of free radicals, particularly superoxide anions and lipid hydroperoxides, which damage the vascular endothelium. Oxidative stress in the systemic circulation in preeclampsia has been explained by free radicals generated by activated neutrophils and the products of lipid peroxidation. Oxidative markers and antioxidants are increased and reduced respectively in the syndrome, including an increase in malondialdehyde and free 8-isoprostane (8-iso-PGF$_2$) (markers of lipid peroxidation) and an excessive reduction in plasma ascorbate (vitamin C) [10]. Although several larger trials are under way to investigate the precise role antioxidant vitamins C and E play in the prevention of preeclampsia, the largest reported so far has concluded that supplementation with combined vitamins C and

E in high-risk patients does not reduce (1) the risk of preeclampsia in nulliparous women, (2) the risk of intrauterine growth restriction, or (3) the risk of death or other serious outcomes in affected infants [11]. Other studies of antioxidant prevention of preeclampsia are still ongoing.

Insulin resistance

Normal pregnancy is a state of insulin resistance, with a doubling in fasting insulin concentrations, likely caused by placental hormones, such as human placental lactogen (hPL) and possibly progesterone and estrogen. It is noteworthy that the many features of preeclampsia, i.e., hypertension, endothelial cell dysfunction, and lipid alterations are important aspects of the insulin resistance syndrome, supporting its potential role in the development of the syndrome; in much the same way as cardiovascular disease in the non-pregnant state.

To further support this hypothesis, it has been demonstrated that plasma levels of glucose after a glucose load are elevated in pregnant women who subsequently develop preeclampsia. Moreover, fasting insulin levels are elevated after an oral glucose tolerance test in women with established disease [12]. Maternal leptin levels, which also correlate with insulin resistance in normal pregnancy, are likewise raised in preeclampsia [13].

In a recent prospective study of pregnant women with normal glucose tolerance and those with gestational diabetes mellitus, TNFα was shown to be a predictor of insulin resistance, emphasizing a close relationship with inflammation [14]. This is further supported by the experimental administration of endotoxin, TNFα and other pro-inflammatory factors, which all induce insulin resistance and hyperlipidemia in animal models.

Dyslipidemia

In normal pregnancy, there is an alteration in lipid profile, including a gestational increase of around 300% in triglycerides (TG) and 25–50% in total cholesterol and an increase in a range of high- and low-density lipoproteins (LDLs). These alterations, which are necessary to fulfill the physiological demands of the fetus, are probably hormonally controlled. In preeclampsia, TG levels are further elevated, particularly in the third trimester, to almost double those of normal pregnancy and LDL levels are concomitantly raised [15]. These alterations, believed to compensate for placenta inefficiencies, may contribute to the endothelial activation of preeclampsia, either directly, through endothelial interactions with TG, or indirectly, through oxidized small dense LDLs, which promote leucocyte–endothelial adhesions, exacerbating the maternal inflammatory response.

Free fatty acids (FFAs) are also raised in preeclampsia, again before the clinical onset of symptoms [16]. These raised levels are major regulators of systemic insulin sensitivity and at the concentrations reported can have a direct impact on vascular endothelial function. Fatty acid synthesis can also be regulated by cytokines, such as TNFα, which inhibits lipogenesis and stimulates lipolysis, proposing an additional role for cytokines in lipid and lipoprotein disturbances.

■ Etiology of preeclampsia

The hypertension associated with preeclampsia generally develops during late pregnancy and remits after delivery or termination, suggesting that the placenta has a critical role. Preeclampsia is often considered a disorder with two components. The first being an as yet unidentified signal that arises from the placenta and is associated with either defective implantation or greater placental mass, such as with hydatidiform moles or twin pregnancies, the second is the aberrant maternal response to this signal, the manifestation of which depends on the maternal genotype and phenotype. This response, which may be amplified by the well characterized physiological and metabolic changes of pregnancy, may also render vascular endothelial cells more sensitive to injury or activation.

Uteroplacental pathology of preeclampsia

It is generally agreed that the underlying cause of preeclampsia is a failure to convert maternal uterine spiral arteries, which supply the developing placenta (see Figure 2.2). In normal pregnancy, invasion of the decidua and myometrium dramatically transforms these uterine vessels, converting them from muscular arteries to wide-mouthed sinusoids. Consequently the vascular supply is transformed from a high-pressure low-flow system to a low-pressure high-flow system to meet the needs of the developing fetus and placenta. The loss of endothelium and muscular layers within these uterine vessels renders them unresponsive to vasomotor stimuli.

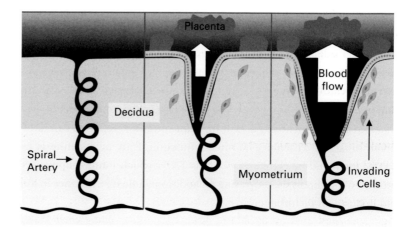

Figure 2.2 Abnormal placentation in preeclampsia. In normal placental development, invasive cells of placental origin invade the maternal uterine spiral arteries (shown in the left panel), transforming them from small-caliber resistance vessels to high-caliber capacitance vessels, capable of providing adequate perfusion to sustain fetal development (right panel). In preeclampsia, placental cell invasion is impaired and the spiral arteries remain as small-caliber resistance vessels (middle panel). This may result in placental underperfusion and/or ischemia.

In preeclampsia, around a half of the necessary decidual spiral arteries undergo these physiological changes and the conversion of their myometrial components fails to occur, resulting in restricted blood flow and the potential for feto-placental hypoxia. In addition, these vessels maintain their muscular coats, and remain sensitive to vasomotor stimuli. This potentially leads to variable oxygenation in the placenta, generating free radicals and oxidative stress. In preeclampsia, typically of increased severity and early-onset phenotype, intraplacental hypoxia and localized ischemia are anticipated from uterine artery Doppler velocimetry, where resistance indices and waveform notching are predictive of impedance to flow. These features of aberrant perfusion and hemodynamics may be confounded by acute atherosis and the formation of intraluminal atherosclerotic plaques, a common feature of untransformed maternal spiral arteries.

It is believed that as a result of hypoperfusion and/or oxidative stress in the placenta, a compensatory mechanism is invoked, which liberates placental factors to overcome discrepancies in blood flow. Ultimately these factors initiate the systemic alterations that culminate in the maternal syndrome; it can therefore be suggested that attenuations in maternal physiology and metabolism as seen in preeclampsia are a placental/fetal-directed response to optimize nutrient flow to the fetus. In this respect a number of circulating pathogenic factors have been considered, including angiogenic agents, cytokines, products of lipid peroxidation, autoantibodies, and placental cellular material and debris.

Circulating angiogenic factors

Several lines of evidence support the hypothesis that the ischemic placenta contributes to endothelial cell dysfunction in the maternal vasculature by inducing an alteration in the balance of circulating levels of angiogenic/anti-angiogenic factors such as vascular endothelial growth factor (VEGF), placental growth factor (PlGF) and soluble fms-like tyrosine kinase-1 (sFlt-1 or soluble VEGF receptor-1 [sVEGFR-1]). Perhaps the most important is sFlt-1, which binds to and inhibits VEGF and PlGF activity. Recent data suggest that circulating concentrations of sFlt-1 presage the clinical symptoms of preeclampsia [17]. Its pathogenic importance has also been highlighted in pregnant rats, where exogenous administration induces a preeclamptic-like state with marked hypertension, proteinuria, and glomerular endotheliosis [18]. Cancer patients treated with a VEGF inhibitor can also develop hypertension and proteinuria [19] supporting this concept, but it remains unclear whether impaired placental perfusion directly liberates sFlt-1 from the human placenta or whether this is a secondary phenomenon. Soluble Flt-1 appears not to directly influence vascular endothelial cells at relevant concentrations, and therefore may have more complex pathogenic activity.

Like sFlt-1, soluble endoglin (a co-receptor for transforming growth factor [TGF]-β1 and -β2), another anti-angiogenic protein, has also been detected in pregnancy and is raised in the maternal circulation two to three months before the clinical onset of preeclampsia. The source of soluble endoglin in this case is the placenta, but again a direct effect on the vascular endothelium remains to be defined.

Lipid peroxides

In normal pregnancy placental cells demonstrate signs of lipoprotein oxidation, i.e., oxidative stress, but this is greatly enhanced in preeclampsia. It is considered that the progressively smaller denser LDLs formed in pregnancy are more prone to oxidative damage during their transient through the placenta [20]. The placental syncytiotrophoblast membrane shows decreased fluidity in preeclampsia, suggestive of lipid peroxidation which may predispose the syncytiotrophoblast to increased deportation and membrane shedding, liberating potentially harmful elements into the maternal circulation (see below). It has also been proposed that there is a greater production of stable oxidative metabolites in the placenta in preeclampsia, such as malondialdehyde and 4-hydroxynonenal, and that these can have a toxic effect, thus contributing to widespread endothelial damage [21].

Inflammation and cytokines

Placental hypoxia, resulting from poor placental perfusion, may predispose to preeclampsia by amplifying the release of inflammatory stimuli into the maternal circulation [6]. Alternatively, the activation of maternal neutrophils during their transit through the placenta could provide a feasible pathway for the transfer of oxidative stress from the placenta to the maternal circulation, through the further liberation of cytokines and reactive oxygen species. In support, leukocytes in the uterine veins are significantly activated relative to the peripheral circulation in preeclampsia [22], whilst elastase-positive cells (a marker of neutrophil activation) are also found in increased numbers in the decidua and placental bed, typically associated with sites of acute atherosis [23].

Tumor necrosis factor-alpha can be directly produced from the human placenta in response to hypoxia and this may, in theory, promote endothelial dysfunction, by directly or competitively acting with maternal free fatty acids, particularly unsaturated FFAs [23]. However, to date analysis of the liberation of TNFα, and other cytokines, IL-6, IL-1α, and IL-1β, from tissues from preeclamptic pregnancies fails to show a significant alteration [24]. This therefore questions the role of the placenta in directly disseminating inflammatory cytokines.

Placental fragments and microparticles

Cellular, subcellular, and molecular debris from the placental surface, the syncytiotrophoblast, is shed into the maternal circulation and is of greater abundance in preeclampsia. It is suggested that these elevations and/or inadequate clearance exaggerates the maternal systemic inflammatory response, beyond that of normal pregnancy [24]. Such material may be significantly elevated in preeclampsia from exaggerated placental cell death or turnover [25]. This suggestion is strengthened by a concomitant increase in circulating cytokeratin and soluble fetal DNA, additional derivatives of the syncytiotrophoblast. This placental-derived material has been shown to be directly damaging to vascular endothelial cells and potentially pro-inflammatory through interactions with circulating phagocytes [26].

Autoantibodies

Women who develop preeclampsia are more likely to develop certain autoantibodies than those of normal pregnancy, and these can still be present even two years following childbirth. Recent studies have shown that women with preeclampsia possess autoantibodies, termed AT1-AAs, that bind to and activate the angiotensin II receptor type 1a (AT1 receptor) [27]. Whether these autoantibodies contribute to the vascular endothelial stress of the condition is unknown. Nevertheless, too much AT1 receptor activation in the presence of autoantibodies is known to cause high blood pressure and inflammation. This has also been demonstrated in pregnant mice after injection with either total immunoglobulin G or affinity-purified AT1-AAs from women with preeclampsia, which demonstrate the main features of the condition, including placental abnormalities and fetal growth restriction [28]. These new studies indicate that preeclampsia may be a pregnancy-induced autoimmune disease and this could have far reaching implications for screening, diagnosis, and therapy.

Genetics

The maternal predisposition to preeclampsia is not the same for all women, and there is undoubtedly a genetic and perhaps environmental component to the syndrome. The evidence for a genetic basis arises from the increased frequency in mothers, daughters, sisters, and granddaughters of women who previously had preeclampsia; in addition there is convincing evidence for a fetal and paternal component to risk [29]. Studies of candidate genes as indicators of susceptibility have highlighted heritable variations in the uteroplacental renin–angiotensin system, as well as other placental genes including *ACVR2* and *STOX1* and those involved in the regulation of placental angiogenesis, e.g., PlGF, VEGF, Flt-1, and endoglin. Some encouraging results have also been obtained in the area of immunogenetics (especially human leukocyte antigen), oxidative stress, and lipid metabolism. Notwithstanding, large-scale multicenter studies, incorporating fetal and maternal genotyping, will be required to truly identify genetic associations.

■ Conclusion and pathogenic model

Normal pregnancy is characterized by mild systemic inflammation, oxidative stress, and alterations in the levels of angiogenic factors and vascular reactivity. These are exacerbated in all hypertensive disorders of pregnancy, ranging from mild gestational hypertension to severe preeclampsia. In the latter, the underlying pathology is thought to be one of relative hypoxia or ischemia of the human placenta with an associated breakdown of compensatory mechanisms, eventually leading to placental and vascular dysfunction.

In the absence of further evidence, a plausible hypothesis for the pathogenesis of preeclampsia is given in Figure 2.3. In these events reduced placental perfusion, as a result of inappropriate placentation (perhaps under genetic, immunological, and environmental control) leads to increased lipid peroxidation and the release of oxygen radicals without counter-regulation by placental or peripheral antioxidants. This hypoxia/oxidative stress may further attenuate placental function but also elicits a maternal, fetal, and/or placental response to optimize nutrient delivery to the fetus.

Currently the link between placental hypoxia, oxidative stress, and maternal vascular dysfunction, the cornerstone of the syndrome, remains elusive but speculated to be a reaction to either placental-derived cell material, shed from the stressed placenta, or humoral factors released into the maternal circulation, such as sFlt-1, soluble endoglin, TNFα, and/or AT1-AA.

The exact mechanism by which these humoral factors induce the widespread activation/dysfunction of the maternal vascular endothelium of the kidney and other organs, causing hypertension, is unknown. Some may be autacoids with direct vasoactive impact, whilst others may perpetuate systemic oxidation, encouraging an inflammatory response in

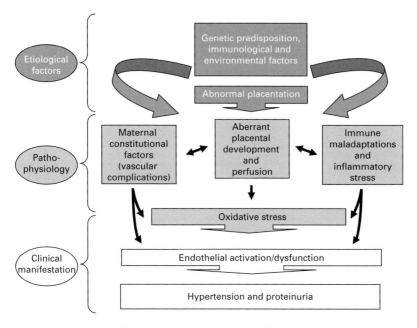

Figure 2.3 The proposed etiology and pathophysiology of preeclampsia.

leukocytes and the endothelium. Ultimately clotting and anticlotting mechanisms are affected, progressing to a hypercoagulatory state, which leads to decreased production of PGI_2 and a simultaneous increase in the vasoconstrictor, thromboxane A_2. A further increase in total peripheral resistance is generated by a reduction in the bioavailability of vasodilators, such as NO, and increase in constrictors, such as reactive oxygen and endothelin-1 (ET-1).

It is envisaged that any preexisting maternal vascular dysfunction is intensified by these placental factors, and this could be responsible for the individual pathologies of the syndrome. The vascular stress test of pregnancy is therefore considered to identify women with a previously unrecognized, but at-risk vascular system. Some women readily tolerate the metabolic and physiological adaptations to pregnancy, even those exaggerated by placental insufficiencies, others however may only partially tolerate these adaptations, resulting in gestational hypertension and mild preeclampsia, whilst others still fail to tolerate these changes and develop severe preeclampsia, with the possibility of eclamptic convulsions.

REFERENCES

1. Barker DJ. Maternal nutrition, fetal nutrition, and disease in later life. *Nutrition* 1997;**13**(9):807–13.

2. Sattar N, Greer IA. Pregnancy complications and maternal cardiovascular risk: opportunities for intervention and screening? *BMJ* 2002;**325**(7356):157–60.

3. Knock GA, Poston L. Bradykinin-mediated relaxation of isolated maternal resistance arteries in normal pregnancy and pre-eclampsia. *Am J Obstet Gynecol* 1996;**175**(6):1668–74.

4. Cockell AP, Poston L. Flow-mediated vasodilatation is enhanced in normal pregnancy but reduced in preeclampsia. *Hypertension* 1997;**30**(2 Pt 1):247–51.

5. Gilbert JS, Ryan MJ, LaMarca BB, *et al.* Pathophysiology of hypertension during preeclampsia: linking placental ischemia with endothelial dysfunction. *Am J Physiol Heart Circ Physiol* 2008;**294**(2):H541–50.

6. Redman CW, Sacks GP, Sargent IL. Preeclampsia: an excessive maternal inflammatory response to pregnancy. *Am J Obstet Gynecol* 1999;**180**(2 Pt 1): 499–506.

7. Sacks GP, Studena K, Sargent K, Redman CW. Normal pregnancy and preeclampsia both produce inflammatory changes in peripheral blood leucocytes akin to those of sepsis. *Am J Obstet Gynecol* 1998;**179**(1):80–6.

8. Rodie VA, Freeman DJ, Sattar N, Greer IA. Pre-eclampsia and cardiovascular disease: metabolic syndrome of pregnancy? *Atherosclerosis* 2004;**175**(2): 189–202.

9. Nadar S, Lip GYH. Platelet activation in the hypertensive disorders of pregnancy. *Expert Opin Investig Drugs* 2004;**13**:523–9.

10. Hubel CA. Oxidative stress in the pathogenesis of preeclampsia. *Proc Soc Exp Biol Med* 1999;**222**(3):222–35.

11. Poston L, Briley AL, Seed PT, Kelly FJ, Shennan AH. Vitamin C and vitamin E in pregnant women at risk for pre-eclampsia (VIP trial): randomised placebo-controlled trial. *Lancet* 2006;**367**(9517):1145–54.

12. Lorentzen B, Birkeland KI, Endresen MJ, Henriksen T. Glucose intolerance in women with preeclampsia. *Acta Obstet Gynecol Scand* 1998;**77**(1):22–7.

13. Laivuori H, Kaaja R, Koistinen H, *et al.* Leptin during and after preeclamptic or normal pregnancy: its relation to serum insulin and insulin sensitivity. *Metabolism* 2000;**49**(2):259–63.

14. Kirwan JP, Hauguel-De Mouzon S, Lepercq J, *et al.* TNF-alpha is a predictor of insulin resistance in human pregnancy. *Diabetes* 2002;**51**(7):2207–13.

15. Sattar N, Bendomir A, Berry C, *et al.* Lipoprotein subfraction concentrations in preeclampsia: pathogenic parallels to atherosclerosis. *Obstet Gynecol* 1997; **89**(3):403–8.

16. Sattar N, Gaw A, Packard CJ, Greer IA. Potential pathogenic roles of aberrant lipoprotein and fatty acid metabolism in pre-eclampsia. *Br J Obstet Gynaecol* 1996;**103**(7):614–20.

17. Levine RJ, Maynard SE, Qian C, *et al.* Circulating angiogenic factors and the risk of preeclampsia. *N Engl J Med* 2004;**350**(7):672–83.

18. Karumanchi SA, Stillman IE. In vivo rat model of preeclampsia. *Methods Mol Med* 2006;**122**:393–9.

19. Yang JC, Haworth L, Sherry RM, *et al.* A randomized trial of bevacizumab, an anti-vascular endothelial growth factor antibody, for metastatic renal cancer. *N Engl J Med* 2003;**349**(5):427–34.

20. Bonet B, Chait A, Gown AM, Knopp RH. Metabolism of modified LDL by cultured human placental cells. *Atherosclerosis* 1995;**112**(2):125–36.

21. Esterbauer H. Cytotoxicity and genotoxicity of lipid-oxidation products. *Am J Clin Nutr* 1993;**57**(5 Suppl):779S–85S; discussion 85S–6S.

22. Mellembakken JR, Aukrust P, Olafsen MK, *et al.* Activation of leucocytes during the uteroplacental passage in preeclampsia. *Hypertension* 2002;**39**(1):155–60.

23. Butterworth BH, Greer IA, Liston WA, Haddad NG, Johnston TA. Immunocyto-chemical localization of neutrophil elastase in term placenta decidua and myometrium in pregnancy-induced hypertension. *Br J Obstet Gynaecol* 1991;**98**(9):929–33.

24. Benyo DF, Smarason A, Redman CW, Sims C, Conrad KP. Expression of inflam-matory cytokines in placentas from women with preeclampsia. *J Clin Endocrinol Metab* 2001;**86**(6):2505–12.

25. Crocker I. Gabor Than Award Lecture 2006: pre-eclampsia and villous tropho-blast turnover: perspectives and possibilities. *Placenta* 2007;**28** Suppl A:S4–13.

26. Abumaree MH, Stone PR, Chamley LW. The effects of apoptotic, deported human placental trophoblast on macrophages: possible consequences for pregnancy. *J Reprod Immunol* 2006;**72**(1–2):33–45.

27. Irani RA, Xia Y. The functional role of the renin-angiotensin system in preg-nancy and preeclampsia. *Placenta* 2008;**29**(9):763–71.

28. Zhou CC, Zhang Y, Irani RA, *et al.* Angiotensin receptor agonistic autoantibo-dies induce pre-eclampsia in pregnant mice. *Nat Med* 2008;**14**(8):855–62.

29. Roberts JM, Cooper DW. Pathogenesis and genetics of pre-eclampsia. *Lancet* 2001;**357**(9249):53–6.

Classification and diagnosis of hypertension in pregnancy

3

Fergus P. McCarthy and Louise C. Kenny

■ Introduction

Hypertensive disorders are a frequently encountered complication of pregnancy and remain a major cause of maternal and perinatal morbidity and mortality [1]. In the United Kingdom the number of maternal deaths from hypertension in pregnancy have fallen steadily over the past few decades, as have the complication rates [2]. The Confidential Enquiry into Stillbirths and Deaths in Infancy report cites one in six stillbirths as occurring in pregnancies complicated by maternal hypertension. Hypertensive disorders vary from mild gestational hypertension to severe preeclampsia and have a number of possible etiologies. Interventions to prevent hypertensive disorders in pregnancy including preeclampsia in the general population have been disappointing and the mainstay of treatment involves close antenatal supervision and timely delivery of mother and baby with a multidisciplinary team approach to prevent deterioration of the condition and subsequent morbidity and mortality [3].

■ Hypertension in pregnancy

Classification of hypertension in pregnancy

The classification of hypertension in pregnancy by Davey and MacGillivray remains the most widely accepted and appropriate classification [4] (Table 3.1).

Hypertension in Pregnancy, ed. Alexander Heazell, Errol R. Norwitz, Louise C. Kenny, and Philip N. Baker. Published by Cambridge University Press. © Cambridge University Press 2010.

Table 3.1 Classification of hypertension in pregnancy

A. New-onset hypertension and/or proteinuria in pregnancy
    1. Gestational hypertension (without proteinuria)
    2. Gestational proteinuria (without hypertension)
    3. Preeclampsia (hypertension with proteinuria)

B. Chronic hypertension and renal disease
    1. Chronic hypertension without proteinuria
    2. Chronic renal disease (proteinuria with or without hypertension)
    3. Chronic hypertension with superimposed preeclampsia (i.e., with new-onset proteinuria in pregnancy)

C. Unclassified
    1. Hypertension and/or proteinuria noted when first presentation is after 20 weeks
    2. As above, when noted for the first time during pregnancy, labor or, puerperium and there are insufficient background data to permit a diagnosis from category A or B above

Source: From: Davey DA, MacGillivray I. The classification and definition of the hypertensive disorders of pregnancy. *Am J Obstet Gynecol* 1988;**158**(4):892–8 [4] with permission from Elsevier.

Women who are hypertensive and pregnant must be subdivided into those with:
- Chronic hypertension
- Pregnancy-induced or gestational hypertension (GH).

Women with GH are subdivided further:
- The majority have non-proteinuric GH, a condition associated with minimal maternal or perinatal morbidity and mortality
- A minority have the major pregnancy complication of preeclampsia.

Diagnosis of hypertension in pregnancy

It is imperative that every effort is made to accurately classify women with hypertension in pregnancy as having chronic hypertension, GH, or preeclampsia because the etiology, management, and prognosis of the three conditions is very different. Appropriate recording of blood pressure is essential for accurate diagnosis and the Royal College of Obstetricians and Gynaecologists study group on preeclampsia recommend the following:
- A mercury or aneroid sphygmomanometer or validated automated device should be used.

- An appropriate cuff size must be used; it is better to use one that is too big than one that is too small.
- The patient should be in a relaxed, quiet environment, preferably after rest, lying at a 45-degree angle or sitting with the cuff at the level of the heart.
- The left or right arm may be used (use the higher value if difference is greater than 10 mmHg).
- Use the dependent arm (lower arm), if in a lateral position [5].
- The first (systolic) and fifth (diastolic) Korotkoff sounds are used to record blood pressure readings; if diastolic is persistently less than 40 mmHg use muffling or fourth sound and make a note [6].

A single blood pressure of 140/90 mmHg or above is not uncommon in pregnancy and was reported in nearly 40% of pregnant women in one study [7]. Therefore, hypertension is defined as a systolic blood pressure ≥ 140 mmHg and/or diastolic blood pressure ≥ 90 mmHg on at least two separate occasions measured at least 6 hours apart. Some clinicians may also define hypertension in pregnancy as a rise in blood pressure from preconception or first-trimester blood pressure values of more than 25 mmHg systolic or 15 mmHg diastolic. It is generally accepted that severe hypertension is confirmed with a diastolic blood pressure ≥ 110 mmHg on two occasions or a systolic blood pressure ≥ 170 mmHg on two occasions. Persistent high blood pressure occurs in approximately 12–22% of pregnancies [8,9].

Once the diagnosis of hypertension has been confirmed urinalysis should be performed to allow appropriate diagnosis. The absence of proteinuria suggests the diagnosis of GH or chronic hypertension.

Gestational hypertension

Gestational hypertension is defined as a systolic blood pressure ≥ 140 mmHg and/or a diastolic blood pressure ≥ 90 mmHg, in the absence of proteinuria, in a previously normotensive pregnant woman at or after 20 weeks of gestation [10]. True non-proteinuric GH does not appear to be associated with an increase in maternal or fetal morbidity. It is unclear whether GH and preeclampsia are different diseases with a similar phenotype or whether GH is a mild or early form of preeclampsia (discussed in Chapter 6). The risk of progression from GH to preeclampsia is approximately 20–30% and therefore increased antenatal surveillance is recommended [11].

Chronic hypertension

Chronic hypertension is defined as hypertension preceding pregnancy. Blood pressure falls slightly in the first and second trimesters. Therefore, women with high blood pressure before the 20th week of pregnancy are assumed to have preexisting or essential hypertension. As many women of reproductive age only present to their healthcare providers for the first time when pregnant, chronic hypertension is often revealed in the first half of pregnancy. Approximately 90% of cases of chronic hypertension are considered to be essential. Secondary causes which account for approximately 10% are listed in Table 3.2 in addition to clinical investigations recommended to assist in the diagnosis of these conditions (discussed in Chapter 7). In women presenting with hypertension in the first half of pregnancy it is important to look for an underlying cause. These investigations should at least include:

- Urine analysis (looking for blood, protein, or glucose)
- Urea and electrolytes
- Renal tract ultrasound.

Women with underlying renal disease are at significantly increased risk of poor pregnancy outcome and require multidisciplinary care. Secondary causes of hypertension are discussed in further detail in Chapter 7.

All pregnant women with a systolic blood pressure of 160 mmHg or more require antihypertensive treatment [2]. Consideration should also be given to initializing treatment at lower pressures if the overall clinical picture suggests rapid deterioration and/or where the development of severe hypertension can be anticipated e.g., co-existing pathology such as systemic lupus erythematosus [12]. Potential antihypertensive agents are discussed in Chapters 5 and 6.

■ Preeclampsia

Introduction

Preeclampsia is a major cause of maternal and perinatal mortality and morbidity worldwide, causing 15% of all direct maternal deaths in the UK and a fivefold increase in perinatal mortality with iatrogenic prematurity being the main cause. It usually occurs during the second half of

Table 3.2 Causes of secondary chronic hypertension and recommended investigative laboratory tests

Etiology	Medical diagnosis	Recommended investigative tests
Idiopathic	Essential hypertension	Diagnosis of exclusion
Vascular disorders	Renovascular hypertension	Renal arteriography, magnetic resonance angiography, computed tomography (CT) angiography, Duplex Doppler ultrasonography
	Aortic coarctation	Echocardiography, Magnetic resonance imaging, CT
Endocrine disorders	Diabetes mellitus	Glucose tolerance test (GTT)
	Hyperthyroidism	Thyroid function tests
	Hypothyroidism	Thyroid function tests
	Pheochromocytoma	24-hour urine catecholamines and metanephrines
	Acromegaly	Growth hormone-dependent circulating molecules, such as IGF-1 and IGFBP-3. Plasma growth hormone levels following GTT
	Cushing's syndrome	24-hour urinary cortisol, low-dose dexamethasone suppression test
	Conn's syndrome (primary aldosteronism)	Elevated plasma aldosterone concentration: plasma renin activity ratio
Renal disorders	Renal failure resulting from:	
	Diabetic nephropathy	
	Reflux nephropathy	
	Chronic glomerulonephritis	
	Nephritic and nephrotic syndrome	
	Polycystic kidney	Renal ultrasound
Connective tissue disorders	Systemic lupus erythematosus	Double-stranded DNA antibodies, anti-smooth muscle antibodies, Antiphospholipid antibodies
	Systemic sclerosis	Autoantibodies including anti-centromere, anti-topoisomerase-I (Scl-70), anti-RNA polymerase, or anti-U3-RNP antibodies are suggestive of systemic sclerosis
	Polyarteritis nodosa	Biopsy of a clinically affected organ
	Rheumatoid disease	Rheumatoid factor

Note: IGF-1, insulin-like growth factor 1; IGFBP-3, insulin-like growth factor binding protein 3.

Table 3.3 Risk factors for preeclampsia

Risk factor	Unadjusted relative risk (95% confidence interval)
Age ≥ 40 years, primiparae	1.68 (1.23–2.29)
Age ≥ 40 years, multiparae	1.96 (1.34–2.87)
Family history	2.90 (1.70–4.93)
Nulliparity	2.91 (1.28–6.61)
Multiple pregnancy	2.93 (2.04–4.21)
Preexisting diabetes	3.56 (2.54–4.99)
Pre-pregnancy body mass index $\geq 35 \text{kg/m}^2$	4.29 (3.52–5.49)
Previous preeclampsia	7.19 (5.85–8.83)
Antiphospholipid syndrome	9.72 (4.34–21.75)

pregnancy and complicates 2–8% of pregnancies. Preeclampsia is twice as common in primigravid women as in women having second or later pregnancies. Women who become pregnant with donor eggs are at increased risk of developing preeclampsia while particular men are at increased risk of fathering a preeclamptic pregnancy. Table 3.3 highlights other risk factors for preeclampsia.

Diagnosis of preeclampsia

Once the diagnosis of hypertension in pregnancy is confirmed as described above, urinalysis must be performed to exclude the more serious diagnosis of preeclampsia. Preeclampsia is defined by the International Society for the Study of Hypertension in Pregnancy as gestational hypertension of at least 140/90 mmHg on two separate occasions measured at least 4 hours apart accompanied by significant proteinuria of at least 300 mg in a 24-hour collection of urine, arising *de novo* after the 20th week of gestation in a previously normotensive woman and resolving completely by the 6th postpartum week [4].

Significant proteinuria is the most important clinical variable predicting both maternal and perinatal outcome. Traditionally, a 24-hour urine collection would be performed and significant proteinuria defined as at least 300 mg protein. An extra benefit of this approach, if creatinine is also measured, is that it allows for the calculation of the glomerular filtration rate from the values of creatinine clearance rate. The 24-hour collection is begun at the usual time that the patient awakens. At that time, the first void is discarded and the exact time noted. Subsequently, all urine voids are collected with the last void timed to finish the collection at exactly the same time the next morning. The time of the final urine specimen should vary by no more than 5 or 10 minutes from the time of starting the collection the previous morning.

A 2+ dipstick measurement may be taken as evidence of proteinuria but there is considerable observer error involved in dipstick urinalysis for proteinuria. Increasingly a spot protein:creatinine ratio is being used in place of a 24-hour urine collection. A protein:creatinine ratio of 0.03 g/mmol appears to be equivalent to 0.3 g protein/24 hours and may be used to check for significant proteinuria. The advantages of using the protein:creatinine ratio over a 24-hour urine collection are that it is far more convenient for the patient, minimizes collection error, and saves time in obtaining results. There is no consensus on the ideal protein:creatinine ratio which will identify significant proteinuria. However, a systematic review of 1214 women performed to assess the diagnostic accuracy of urinary spot protein:creatinine ratio for proteinuria in hypertensive pregnant women concluded that the spot urine ratio had a sensitivity of 83.6% (95% confidence interval [CI], 77.5–89.7) and a specificity of 76.3% (95% CI, 72.6–80.0) using cutoffs ranging from 0.15 to 0.50 grams of protein per gram of creatinine [13].

In addition to presenting with hypertension and significant proteinuria, patients with preeclampsia may also become symptomatic and present with any of the following symptoms; headache, epigastric or right upper quadrant pain, visual disturbances, and nausea or vomiting.

Prediction of preeclampsia

Although multiple risk factors have been described for the development of preeclampsia (Table 3.3) our ability to screen for and predict the occurrence and onset of preeclampsia is poor. The use of uterine artery Doppler velocimetry for prediction of preeclampsia has been extensively investigated but has been shown to have consistently low sensitivity and a high false positive rate [14]. As a result its use is not recommended in routine practice. Other potential screening tests include measurement of urinary and plasma angiogenic factors (vascular endothelial growth factor, placental growth factor, soluble endoglin [sEng] and soluble fms-like tyrosine kinase-1 [sFlt-1]), measurement of plasma uric acid levels or measurement of maternal serum markers such as alpha-fetoprotein, human chorionic gonadotropin, inhibin A, and activin A. However, to date there is no recommended screening tool for the prediction of preeclampsia.

■ Postpartum hypertension

Blood pressure rises progressively over the first five postnatal days, peaking on day's three to six after delivery. Research has focused on the antenatal complications, for both mother and baby, and the risks and benefits of administering antihypertensive therapy prior to delivery [15]. There is very little information on how best to manage postpartum hypertension, regardless of type or severity, to optimize maternal safety and minimize hospital stay. The true prevalence of postpartum hypertension is difficult to ascertain, but the importance of monitoring women in the puerperium was highlighted by the Confidential Enquiry into Maternal and Child Health (CEMACH), in which roughly 10% of maternal deaths due to a hypertensive disorder of pregnancy occurred in the postpartum period. Women with postpartum hypertension may also experience longer hospital stays and possibly, heightened anxiety about their recovery.

In most cases of GH and preeclampsia there is a rapid and complete resolution within six weeks of delivery of the fetus. Patients requiring antihypertensives can be weaned off slowly and medications should not be stopped suddenly as there may often be a rebound hypertension resulting in a prolonged inpatient stay.

Postnatal follow-up

Women who have had hypertension during pregnancy should be followed up postpartum to ensure full resolution of their hypertension. Women who have suffered from preeclampsia during their pregnancy should be educated regarding their increased risk of development of cardiovascular disease, renal disease, and cardiovascular risk factors for several years following pregnancy and regular blood pressure checks with their general practitioner should be recommended [16,17]. Women with severe preeclampsia have an increased risk of recurrence in their next pregnancy but the disorder is generally less severe and manifests two to three weeks later than in the first pregnancy. Women with a history of severe early-onset preeclampsia, especially if associated with intrauterine growth restriction or stillbirth, should be screened for antiphospholipid syndrome, hyperhomocysteinuria, factor V Leiden mutation, protein S, protein C, and antithrombin III deficiency and the implications of positive test results discussed with the patient.

Women with essential hypertension should be encouraged to present for preconceptual counseling as antihypertensive medications such as angiotensin converting enzyme inhibitors are contraindicated in pregnancy and should be changed preconceptually. The use of low-dose aspirin in women with chronic hypertension moderately reduces the risk of developing superimposed preeclampsia, intrauterine growth retardation, and perinatal death, and should be offered to all women at an early booking visit. The findings from the CLASP trial do not support routine treatment with aspirin of all women at risk of preeclampsia [18].

■ Conclusion

Hypertensive disorders are one of the commonest complications of pregnancy and may be associated with significant maternal and fetal morbidity and mortality. Although the etiology of these disorders is becoming increasingly better understood interventions to predict and prevent hypertensive disorders of pregnancy have had poor results. The mainstay of treatment remains the use of antihypertensive medications, the use of magnesium sulfate in the prevention of eclampsia and multidisciplinary input to ensure a timely delivery.

REFERENCES

1. Khan KS, Wojdyla D, Say L, Gulmezoglu AM, Van Look PF. WHO analysis of causes of maternal death: a systematic review. *Lancet* 2006;**367**(9516):1066–74.
2. Lewis GE. (ed.) The Confidential Enquiry into Maternal and Child Health (CEMACH). *Saving Mothers' Lives: reviewing maternal deaths to make motherhood safer–2003–2005.* The Seventh Report on Confidential Enquiries into Maternal Deaths in the United Kingdom. London, CEMACH, 2007.
3. Sibai BM. Prevention of preeclampsia: a big disappointment. *Am J Obstet Gynecol* 1998;**179**(5):1275–8.
4. Davey DA, MacGillivray I. The classification and definition of the hypertensive disorders of pregnancy. *Am J Obstet Gynecol* 1988;**158**(4):892–8.
5. Kinsella SM. Effect of blood pressure instrument and cuff side on blood pressure reading in pregnant women in the lateral recumbent position. *Int J Obstet Anesth* 2006;**15**(4):290–3.
6. Royal College of Obstetricians and Gynaecologists. *The Management of Severe Pre-Eclampsia/Eclampsia, Green Top Guideline 10A.* London, RCOG Press, 2006.

7. Plouin PF, Breart G, Rabarison Y, *et al.* [Incidence and fetal impact of hypertension in pregnancy: study of 2996 pregnancies]. *Arch Mal Coeur Vaiss* 1982;**75** Spec No:5–7.

8. Levine RJ, Hauth JC, Curet LB, *et al.* Trial of calcium to prevent preeclampsia. *N Engl J Med* 1997;**337**(2):69–76.

9. Knight M, Duley L, Henderson-Smart DJ, King JF. Antiplatelet agents for preventing and treating pre-eclampsia. *Cochrane Database Syst Rev* 2000(2): CD000492.

10. Sibai BM. Diagnosis and management of gestational hypertension and preeclampsia. *Obstet Gynecol* 2003;**102**(1):181–92.

11. Saudan P, Brown MA, Buddle ML, Jones M. Does gestational hypertension become pre-eclampsia? *Br J Obstet Gynaecol* 1998;**105**(11):1177–84.

12. Martin JN, Jr., Thigpen BD, Moore RC, *et al.* Stroke and severe preeclampsia and eclampsia: a paradigm shift focusing on systolic blood pressure. *Obstet Gynecol* 2005;**105**(2):246–54.

13. Cote AM, Brown MA, Lam E, *et al.* Diagnostic accuracy of urinary spot protein: creatinine ratio for proteinuria in hypertensive pregnant women: systematic review. *BMJ* 2008;**336**(7651):1003–6.

14. Cnossen JS, Morris RK, ter Riet G, *et al.* Use of uterine artery Doppler ultrasonography to predict pre-eclampsia and intrauterine growth restriction: a systematic review and bivariable meta-analysis. *CMAJ.* 2008;**178**(6):701–11.

15. Altman D, Carroli G, Duley L, *et al.* Do women with pre-eclampsia, and their babies, benefit from magnesium sulphate? The Magpie Trial: a randomised placebo-controlled trial. *Lancet* 2002;**359**(9321):1877–90.

16. Wilson BJ, Watson MS, Prescott GJ, *et al.* Hypertensive diseases of pregnancy and risk of hypertension and stroke in later life: results from cohort study. *BMJ* 2003;**326**(7394):845.

17. Smith GC, Pell JP, Walsh D. Pregnancy complications and maternal risk of ischaemic heart disease: a retrospective cohort study of 129,290 births. *Lancet* 2001;**357**(9273):2002–6.

18. CLASP: a randomised trial of low-dose aspirin for the prevention of pre-eclampsia among 9364 pregnant women. CLASP(Collaborative Low-dose Aspirin Study in Pregnancy) Collaborative Group. *Lancet* 1994;**343** (8898):619–29.

Screening for hypertensive disorders of pregnancy

4

Sarosh Rana, S. Ananth Karumanchi,
and Errol R. Norwitz

■ Introduction

Preeclampsia, characterized by new-onset of hypertension, proteinuria, and often, but not invariably, non-dependent edema after gestational week 20, affects 3–5% of all pregnancies, and is a major cause of maternal, fetal, and neonatal morbidity and mortality worldwide [1]. Preeclampsia may also be accompanied by pathological manifestations in other organ systems, such as microangiopathic hemolytic anemia, liver abnormalities, and central nervous system symptomatology (including convulsions, i.e., eclampsia). It can be superimposed on another hypertensive disorder, and it is the women with both multi-system manifestation and superimposed disease who suffer the greatest morbidity.

The cause of preeclampsia remains obscure, although more and more evidence is accruing to support the hypotheses that the placenta plays a crucial role. Of interest, in this respect, the disease happens only in the presence of pregnancy, usually resolves rapidly after delivery of the placenta, and preeclampsia and eclampsia can occur in molar pregnancies without the presence of a fetus [2]. Some describe preeclampsia's etiology as a two-step process, the first, an asymptomatic stage (placental), involves abnormal placentation, which then is followed by placental elaboration of soluble factors that enter the maternal circulation and

Hypertension in Pregnancy, ed. Alexander Heazell, Errol R. Norwitz, Louise C. Kenny, and Philip N. Baker. Published by Cambridge University Press. © Cambridge University Press 2010.

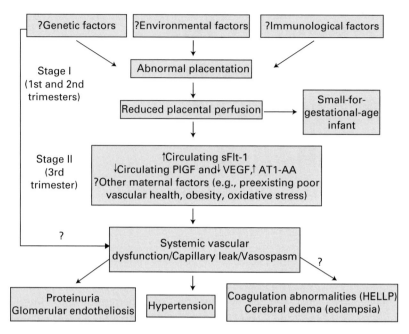

Figure 4.1 Schematic representation of the pathophysiological processes involved in preeclampsia. ATI-AA, angiotensin II receptor 1 autoantibodies; HELLP, hemolysis, elevated liver enzymes, and low platelets; PIGF, placental growth factor; sFlt-1, soluble Fms-like tyrosine kinase-1; VEGF, vascular endothelial growth factor.

cause widespread endothelial dysfunction [3] (see Figure 4.1). At particular risk are pregnant women with disorders that make them susceptible to assaults on their vasculature (i.e., women with chronic hypertension or with metabolic disorders such as diabetes, those who are obese, or have had preeclampsia in a previous pregnancy).

Delineation of a reliable and safe screening test for preeclampsia has been an investigator's dream for many decades, and an extensive systematic review of most of these tests was published in 2004 [4]. The authors analyzed 87 out of 7191 potentially relevant articles (211 369 women) that described a variety of biophysical and biochemical tests, assessing their usefulness in predicting preeclampsia. The authors concluded that there were no clinically useful screening tests to predict the development of preeclampsia [4]. The review did note moderate predictive accuracy for anticardiolipin antibodies, the presence of bilateral notching on uterine artery Doppler ultrasonography, and urinary kallikrein (a test not readily available in clinical laboratories). This review, however, did not consider the predictive power of combining the results of different tests, nor did it undertake analyses of a just-emerging literature on the ability of anti- and pro-angiogenic proteins to predict the disease, as this literature was then in its infancy.

This chapter will focus on ultrasound markers (uterine artery Doppler velocimetry) and emerging literature on serum markers (mainly placental protein-13 [PP-13] and angiogenic proteins) as methods to predict preeclampsia.

■ Uterine artery Doppler velocimetry

The primary mechanism for preeclampsia is being proposed as failure of adequate trophoblast invasion into the maternal spiral arteries. This results in increased vascular resistance in the uteroplacental unit which leads to decreased perfusion of the placenta and subsequently results in fetal growth restriction and/or preeclampsia [5]. Uterine artery Doppler ultrasound is a non-invasive method to examine the uteroplacental circulation that provides indirect evidence of this process and has consequently been proposed as a predictive test for preeclampsia [6]. Uterine artery Doppler ultrasonography may be performed via the transvaginal or transabdominal route in the first or second trimester. The uterine artery is identified with the use of color Doppler ultrasonography and then pulsed-wave Doppler ultrasonography is used to obtain waveforms. The increase in flow resistance within the uterine arteries results in an abnormal waveform pattern, which is represented by either an increased resistance index or pulsatility index (PI) or by the persistence of unilateral or bilateral diastolic notching (see Figure 4.2). Several flow velocity waveforms, single or combined, have been investigated for the prediction of preeclampsia. There are a number of studies involving use of Doppler ultrasound alone or in combination with serum markers to predict preeclampsia.

A recently published meta-analysis (2008) looked at the accuracy of 15 different uterine artery Doppler indices in the first and second trimesters for prediction of preeclampsia [7]. It included 74 studies (69 cohort studies, 3 randomized controlled trials, and 2 case-control studies) in which uterine artery Doppler ultrasonography had been used, calculated the sensitivity and specificity for each study, and pooled the results of studies with similar Doppler indices, outcomes, and patient risk. This analysis

(a)

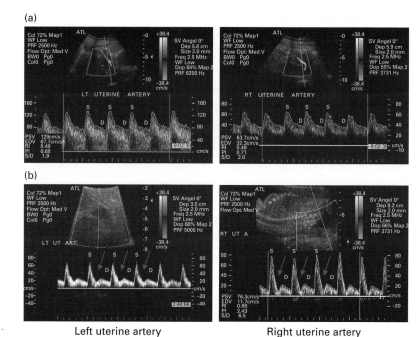

(b)

Left uterine artery   Right uterine artery

Figure 4.2 (a) Uterine artery Doppler blood flow in normal pregnancy demonstrating no diastolic notch. (b) Uterine artery notching in a case of preeclampsia (marked with arrows). See plate section for color version.

concluded that an increased PI with notching in the second trimester best predicted overall preeclampsia in low-risk patients (positive likelihood ratio [LR], 7.5; 95% confidence interval [CI], 5.4–10.2; and negative LR, 0.59; 95% CI, 0.47–0.71) and in high-risk patients (positive LR, 21.0; 95% CI, 5.5–80.5; and negative LR, 0.82; 95% CI, 0.72–0.93). In one prospective study by Pilalis *et al.*, 878 consecutive women who presented for a routine prenatal ultrasound examination at 11–14 weeks underwent uterine artery Doppler interrogation [8]. The mean PI of the uterine arteries was calculated. Maternal serum samples for pregnancy-associated plasma protein-A (PAPP-A) were also assayed. Along with maternal history, these measurements were compared in their ability to predict adverse outcome including preeclampsia. This study found that the mean uterine artery PI $\geq$ 95th percentile and PAPP-A $\leq$ 10th percentile each identified 23% of the women that went on to develop preeclampsia. Independent predictors for subsequent development of preeclampsia were increased mean uterine artery PI $\geq$ 95th percentile (odds ratio [OR], 2.76; 95% CI, 1.11–6.81) and maternal history of preeclampsia/hypertension (OR, 50.54; 95% CI, 10.52–242.73). Another study by Spencer *et al.* looked at maternal serum PP-13 and PAPP-A at 11^{+0} to 13^{+6} weeks of gestation alone or in combination with second-trimester uterine artery PI measured by Doppler velocimetry in predicting those women who will develop preeclampsia [9]. They found that median PP-13 and PAPP-A were lower while uterine artery PI was higher in patients who developed early preeclampsia (delivery < 35 weeks). Combining PP-13 and PI using logistic regression analysis yielded an area under the curve of 0.90 (95% CI, 0.84–0.96; $P < 0.001$) and a sensitivity of 0.79 in the early cases. Pregnancy-associated plasma protein-A with PI gave an area under the curve of 0.82 (95% CI, 0.76–0.90; $P < 0.001$) and a sensitivity of 0.76 in all cases. Combining PAPP-A with PP-13 and PI did not add significantly to the sensitivity. They concluded that first-trimester PP-13 levels might be useful in predicting preeclampsia and early preeclampsia, and the accuracy of the method increases when coupled with second-trimester Doppler PI measurement.

Similar to the above studies, uterine artery Doppler is also studied in combination with angiogenic proteins (discussed later in the chapter) to predict preeclampsia. Crispi *et al.* [10] investigated potential differences in the prediction of early- versus late-onset preeclampsia and/or intrauterine growth restriction (PE/IUGR) by second-trimester uterine artery Doppler examination, and measurement of maternal serum placental growth factor (PlGF) and soluble fms-like tyrosine kinase-1 (sFlt-1). Uterine artery mean PI and maternal serum PlGF and sFlt-1 levels were measured at 24 weeks of gestation in 76 healthy pregnant women and 38 cases of PE/IUGR, of which 19 were defined as early onset (< 32 weeks). They found that, for a specificity of 95%, the sensitivities of uterine artery mean PI, PlGF, and sFlt-1 for early-onset PE/IUGR were 47.4%, 84.4%, and 36.8%, respectively. When combining uterine artery Doppler with PlGF, the sensitivity for identifying early-onset PE/IUGR was 89.5% with a specificity of 95%. Conversely, the sensitivity for late-onset PE/IUGR was below 11% for all parameters analyzed. In a similar study, Stepan *et al.* [11] looked at 77 second-trimester pregnant women with abnormal uterine perfusion and measured serum soluble endoglin (sEng) and sFlt-1. They found that adverse pregnancy outcome was associated with higher sEng levels in the second trimester. Soluble endoglin was highest in those pregnancies with early-onset preeclampsia. Combined analysis of sEng and sFlt-1 was able to predict early-onset preeclampsia with a sensitivity of 100% and a specificity of 93.3%. They concluded that concurrent measurement of uterine perfusion and angiogenic factors allows a highly efficient prediction of early-onset preeclampsia. However, this study was done in a high-risk group only as all women had abnormal uterine artery Doppler measurements.

Doppler velocimetry is non-invasive and thus acceptable to patients. However, it is highly specialized, both in terms of the equipment required and operator expertise. In industrialized countries, Doppler assessment could be fairly easily performed at the time of a detailed anatomy scan at 18–20 weeks' gestation. However, in developing countries, it would be difficult to introduce this test into routine antenatal practice as a screening tool.

Most of the studies looking at the utility of uterine artery Doppler ultrasound to predict preeclampsia have been done in the mid to late second trimester. There are now multiple studies looking at abnormal serum analyte profiles in the first trimester and the prediction of preeclampsia (as discussed later in the chapter). Consequently, future studies on the utility of uterine artery Doppler velocimetry to identify women at risk of developing preeclampsia (either alone or in combination with serum analyte measurements) will have to focus on the first trimester if they are to have any future clinical utility.

■ Serum markers

Current obstetric practice uses first- and second-trimester maternal serum levels of the β-subunit of human chorionic gonadotropin (β-hCG), alpha-fetoprotein (AFP), unconjugated estriol, inhibin A, PAPP-A, and activin A to screen pregnancies for fetal aneuploidy, neural tube defects, and other fetal abnormalities. Since the results of these tests are available in the early second trimester, it has been proposed that they may be useful also as predictive tests for other pregnancy-related disorders that are characterized by generalized placental dysfunction. To this end, several groups have evaluated the use of these feto-placental proteins for predicting the risk of preeclampsia. Overall, the results of these studies suggest that these markers have very limited predictive accuracy for preeclampsia.

Placental protein-13

Placental protein-13 is a member of the galectin family expressed predominantly by the placenta (specifically by the syncytiotrophoblast), which is thought to be involved in implantation and maternal artery remodeling [12]. Preliminary data suggested that maternal serum PP-13 concentrations are significantly reduced during the first trimester among women who subsequently develop preeclampsia, particularly early-onset preeclampsia. The mechanisms responsible for this reduction have not been determined. Nicolaides *et al.* published a case-control study indicating that patients who developed preeclampsia requiring delivery before 34 weeks of gestation (n = 10) had a lower median PP-13 serum concentration than normotensive controls at 11–14 weeks' gestation [13]. The sensitivity was 90% and the specificity 88%; positive and negative LR were 7.5 and 0.1, respectively.

In a similar nested case–control study, Chafetz *et al.* reported that the median first-trimester serum PP-13 levels were significantly lower among women who had preeclampsia (n = 47) compared with normotensive control subjects (n = 290) [14]. Using a cutoff of 0.38 MoM, the sensitivity was 79% and the specificity 90%; positive and negative LR were 7.9 and 0.2, respectively. Recently, Romero *et al.* reported a case–control study that included 50 women with preeclampsia and 250 with normal pregnancies [15]. Serum PP-13 concentration in the first trimester was significantly lower in women who developed preterm and early-onset preeclampsia than in those with normal pregnancies. At 80% specificity, a cutoff of 0.39 MoM had sensitivity of only 36% for all cases of preeclampsia, 24% for severe preeclampsia (n = 21), and 13% for mild preeclampsia at term (n = 16). Nevertheless, the sensitivities for early-onset preeclampsia (n = 6) and preterm preeclampsia (n = 13) were 100% and 85%, respectively.

In conclusion, maternal serum first-trimester PP-13 appears to be a promising test for the prediction of preeclampsia, mainly early-onset preeclampsia. Nevertheless, additional studies are required to determine whether the results reported from case–control studies can be replicated prospectively in large populations.

Circulating angiogenic factors in the pathogenesis of preeclampsia

There are a host of recent studies looking at the role of angiogenic proteins in the pathogenesis of preeclampsia [16–20]. These studies have established new insights into the mechanisms of several of the disease's major phenotypes (see Chapter 2 for a summary of the pathogenesis of preeclampsia). The findings in these cited studies have led to an extremely plausible hypothesis that the clinical manifestations of preeclampsia result, in part, from an imbalance between circulating pro-angiogenic and anti-angiogenic factors in the maternal circulation. The two anti-angiogenic factors implicated are soluble vascular endothelial growth factor receptor-1 (sVEGFR1, also referred to as sFlt-1) and sEng, whose levels are elevated in women with preeclampsia, while the pro-angiogenic proteins, whose circulating concentrations (free levels) are reduced in women with the disease, include vascular endothelial growth factor (VEGF) and PlGF.

Vascular endothelial growth factor, an endothelial-specific mitogen, plays a key role in promoting angiogenesis [21,22]. Its activities are mediated primarily by interaction with two high-affinity receptor tyrosine kinases, VEGFR-1 (Flt-1) and VEGFR-2 (kinase-insert domain region [KDR]/Flk1), which are selectively expressed on the vascular endothelial cell surface. The VEGFR1 has two isoforms: a transmembranous isoform and a soluble isoform (sVEGFR1 or sFlt-1). The soluble isoform arises from a transcriptional variant resulting in a truncated mRNA that lacks the cytoplasmic and transmembrane domain but contains the ligand-binding domain [23]. Thus, sFlt-1 can antagonize the biological activity of VEGF in the maternal circulation by binding to it and preventing its interaction with its endogenous receptors. Soluble Flt1 also binds and antagonizes PlGF, another member of the VEGF family produced almost exclusively by the placenta. Soluble Flt1 is elevated during clinical preeclampsia and in the weeks preceding clinical symptoms. The elevated levels of sFlt-1 have been associated with a fall in free PlGF and VEGF in the maternal circulation. Furthermore, elevating sFlt-1 levels in pregnant rodents appears to recreate hypertension, proteinuria, and glomerular endotheliosis, all hallmarks of preeclampsia [17].

Soluble endoglin, another anti-angiogenic protein, is a transforming growth factor (TGF)-β1 co-receptor. The putative role of this protein in producing a preeclampsia phenotype was predicated based on the hypothesis that sEng might impair TGF-β1 binding to its cell surface receptors and thereby decrease endothelial nitric oxide (NO) signaling. Nitric oxide, in turn, is known to act at a cellular level and have potent vasodilatory properties. Moreover, it was recently demonstrated that sEng is produced by the placenta, is present in high concentrations in the sera of pregnant women, is elevated in women with preeclampsia, and its levels appear to correlate with disease severity [24]. Administration of both sFlt-1 and sEng using an adenoviral expression system in rats produces a severe preeclampsia-like disorder with hypertension; proteinuria; glomerular endotheliosis; features of hemolysis, elevated liver enzymes, and low platelets (HELLP) syndrome; and small-for-gestational-age (SGA) pups [25].

The evidence implicating sFlt-1 and sEng in the pathogenesis of preeclampsia comes from the measurement of these anti-angiogenic proteins in the circulation of women with confirmed preeclampsia, from in vitro studies using sera from preeclamptic women, and from animal models of preeclampsia. The initial observations that placental expression and serum levels of sFlt-1 are increased during preeclampsia compared with normotensive pregnancies have since been confirmed by several groups [16–18,26]. Other studies have shown that levels of sFlt-1 are positively correlated with gestational age [18,27,28]. Clinically, circulating sFlt-1 levels have been observed to be directly proportional to the severity of proteinuria, but inversely correlated with platelet counts, gestational age, and neonatal birthweight adjusted for gestational age [27]. In women with preeclampsia, circulating levels of sFlt-1 are higher in those with early-onset disease (< 37 weeks) [18,27], more severe disease [17,18,27], and SGA neonates [18,28]. Decreased circulating levels of free VEGF and PlGF, and decreased urinary PlGF have also been demonstrated in women with preeclampsia [29–31]. In contrast, clinical data on sEng in preeclampsia are limited. Two recent studies from a single group have attempted to elucidate the role of sEng in preeclampsia, showing that sEng is elevated in the sera of preeclamptic individuals, correlates with disease severity, and falls after delivery [24,25]. One of the reports suggests that sEng alterations in the maternal circulation pre-date the onset of clinical symptoms of preeclampsia by several months [24]. There are additional data suggesting that elevated circulating levels of sFlt-1 and sEng and reduced levels of PlGF in the mid-trimester may also be evident in pregnancies that later develop hypertension and placental abruption [32,33].

Ability of angiogenic proteins to predict preeclampsia

In preeclampsia, levels of sFlt-1 are higher than normotensive controls at the time of clinical disease. In a cross-sectional nested cohort study using stored samples from a previous clinical trial, Levine and colleagues confirmed that circulating sFlt-1 levels were significantly higher in women with preeclampsia than in gestational age-matched normotensive controls [18]. They also showed that levels of this anti-angiogenic protein were significantly elevated five weeks before the detection of hypertension and proteinuria [18]. While the data from Levine and colleagues were presented primarily as arithmetic means, other investigators have now confirmed these observations using more sophisticated statistical analysis, such as multiples of median. Investigators have measured sFlt-1 levels longitudinally throughout gestation in normal pregnancies and pregnancies that subsequently developed preeclampsia, and reported that sFlt-1 levels are elevated throughout gestation in the circulation of pregnant women destined to develop preeclampsia, and that a significant difference is typically detectable five to six weeks before the disease presents clinically [19,34,35]. However, there is only one published study that measured angiogenic protein levels in early pregnancy. Wathen and colleagues measured sFlt-1 levels at 12–15 weeks and 16–20 weeks in pregnant women who went on to develop preeclampsia or IUGR along with a cohort of uncomplicated normotensive controls. The authors found that an elevated sFlt-1 level at 16–20 weeks is associated with an increased risk of preeclampsia (OR, 2.1; 95% CI, 0.8–5.6) or severe preeclampsia (OR, 4.1; 95% CI, 1.1–15.6). In addition, sFlt-1 concentrations decreased by 15% from first to second sample in controls but not in preeclamptic women [36]. These observations suggest that sequential changes in one or more pro-/ anti-angiogenic factor may be more important than the measured absolute values. Similar findings were reported by Rana *et al.* [37] and Vatten *et al.* [38] demonstrating that longitudinal changes in the levels of circulating angiogenic factors differ in pregnancies destined to develop preeclampsia. For example, a small increase in PlGF and a large increase in sFlt-1 are strong predictors of preeclampsia [38]. Similarly, women who go on to develop early-onset preeclampsia have a pronounced increase in circulating sFlt-1 and sEng levels between the first and second trimesters [37].

In 2006, Levine and colleagues published results of a nested case–control study of healthy nulliparous women in which they measured levels of angiogenic factors (sFlt-1, sEng, and PlGF) in stored sera from the Calcium for Pre-eclampsia Prevention trial [24]. The authors analyzed three gestational age windows: 13–20 weeks, 21–32 weeks, and 33–42 weeks. Included were sera from 72 women who had preterm preeclampsia (< 37 weeks), 120 with term preeclampsia (≥ 37 weeks), 120 with gestational hypertension, 120 who delivered SGA infants but remained normotensive, and 120 with uncomplicated gestations (normotensive controls). Soluble Eng levels were significantly elevated at 17–20 weeks in women destined to develop preterm preeclampsia compared with normotensive controls, and significantly elevated at 25–28 weeks when the disorder developed at term. Of importance too was the observation that sEng levels were not markedly elevated in early or mid-pregnancy in those women destined to develop gestational hypertension or in normotensive women who went on to deliver SGA infants. Finally, the authors examined the risk among women with high or low (highest or lower quartiles) sEng levels and/or sFlt-1/PlGF ratios in serum obtained at 21–32 weeks of gestation. They found that the risk of preeclampsia was significantly elevated among women with both high sEng levels and elevated sFlt-1/PlGF ratios (adjusted OR for preterm preeclampsia, 31.6; 95% CI, 10.7–93.4; and for term preeclampsia, 30.8; 95% CI, 10.8–87.6) as compared with only one abnormal value.

Another promising strategy is urine screening with PlGF assay followed by blood confirmation with sFlt-1/PlGF. In the absence of glomerular damage, sFlt-1 is thought to be too large a molecule to be filtered into the urine, whereas PlGF is readily filtered and can thus be measured and used as a potential predictive test. In a nested case–control study by Levine *et al.*, urinary PlGF was measured in 120 normotensive controls and women who subsequently developed preeclampsia [30]. This study found that low levels of PlGF in the urine at mid-gestation was strongly associated with the subsequent development of preterm preeclampsia. The adjusted OR for the risk of developing preeclampsia < 37 weeks in those women who had urinary PlGF levels in the lowest quartile of control concentrations ($< 118\,\mathrm{pg/mL}$) at 21–32 weeks' gestation was 22.5 compared with all other quartiles.

Of note, the above-cited article [30], although exciting and promising, is retrospective and cross-sectional in study design, and involved the use of stored sera and urine from a study performed over ten years ago. Indeed, its limitations are similar to those noted in a recent systematic review of the use of angiogenic factors to predict preeclampsia [39], which was completed prior to the publication of Levine and colleagues [24] and therefore failed to include any references relating to sEng. The authors of the systematic review noted that most studies were retrospective, that there was considerable heterogeneity among published reports likely due to differences in the gestational windows under investigation and in the inclusion and exclusion criteria used in each of the studies, and that there were differences in the serum analytes being studied and in the storage conditions [39]. There were also considerable differences in the way different laboratories reported the results. The authors underscored the need for additional prospective observational data, and pleaded for standardization of operational procedures in future studies including the importance of assessing imprecision, inaccuracy, linearity, and minimum detectable dose for each assay. They added that the performance of each assay should be confirmed using internal and external quality controls. Finally, the authors noted that this systematic review had formed the basis of the World Health Organization planning phase of the Global Program to Conquer Preeclampsia and its decision to embark on a large prospective observational study in the developing world. Indeed, just such a study was started in late 2006 in six countries (Argentina, Columbia, India, Thailand, Switzerland, and Italy) with a view to measuring sFlt-1, sEng, and PlGF levels longitudinally in blood and urine in approximately 10 000 high- and low-risk women.

Recently, several isoforms of sFlt-1 have been demonstrated to be produced by the placenta [40]. One of these isoforms (referred to as sFlt-1–14) is expressed only in humans and other primates [41]. Soluble Flt1–14 differs from sFlt-1 in that it lacks the C-terminal 31 amino acids and instead contains an additional intron (intron 14) in the C-terminus that codes for a unique 28 amino acids. Assays to measure this specific sFlt-1 isoform in preeclampsia are currently ongoing. Most recently, Bills and co-workers reported that $VEGF_{165}b$, an alternative splice variant of VEGF pre-mRNA, is upregulated in the maternal circulation in normal pregnancy, but that this increase in $VEGF_{165}b$ is delayed or diminished in women who develop preeclampsia [42]. They showed also that women with low $VEGF_{165}b$ levels in the maternal circulation had higher concentrations of sFlt-1 and sEng, which further increased their risk for developing preeclampsia. The authors concluded that low $VEGF_{165}b$ may be an additional independent risk factor for preeclampsia, and that this protein could serve as an early marker for the disease.

Other biomarkers in preeclampsia

Additional studies have identified high titers of anti-angiotensin II receptor autoantibodies (AT1-AA) in women with preeclampsia [43]. These AT1-AA, like angiotensin II itself, may lead to the production of large amounts of tissue factor by endothelial cells which, in turn, could adversely affect trophoblast implantation and placentation. Indeed, Xia *et al.* reported that AT1-AA decreased the invasiveness of immortalized human trophoblast cells using an in vitro invasion assay [44]. Moreover, studies from Zhou *et al.* suggest that AT1-AA recovered from the circulation of women with preeclampsia can replicate the key features of preeclampsia in pregnant mice with an associated increase in circulating levels of both sFlt-1 and sEng [45]. The effects of these antibodies can be blocked with losartan, a pharmacological AT1 receptor antagonist, or by an antibody-neutralizing peptide [46]. Present not only during pregnancy, AT1-AA appear to be increased also in patients with malignant renovascular hypertension and vascular rejection [46]. However, the presence of antiAT1-AA cannot adequately explain the suppression of aldosterone production noted in preeclampsia [47]. In summary, AT1-AA may be one of several insults that can contribute to the placental damage that is proximally linked to the production of anti-angiogenic factors. More research is needed to determine whether measurement of AT1-AA can be used as a predictive marker for early-onset preeclampsia.

Other proteins in the maternal circulation have been investigated as predictive markers of preeclampsia including asymmetric dimethylarginine (ADMA), an endogenous inhibitor of endothelial NO synthase. In a recent study by Speer *et al.*, maternal ADMA concentrations were elevated at mid-pregnancy and remained elevated at delivery in women who later developed preeclampsia as compared with normotensive controls [48]. In another study, uterine artery Doppler velocimetry was assessed at 23–25 weeks' gestation along with measurements of serum ADMA. Women with evidence of high resistance in their placental circulation were at increased risk of developing preeclampsia and/or IUGR, and these same women also had elevated serum concentrations of ADMA [49].

More recently, in a large prospective clinical study involving nearly 8000 subjects, Poon *et al.* demonstrated that a combination of angiogenic factors (PlGF), PAPP-A, and uterine artery Doppler velocimetry in the first trimester can predict the subsequent development of early-onset preeclampsia with a sensitivity of 93% at a 5% false positive rate [50]. These data suggest that combinations of biomarkers may allow clinicians to more accurately predict early-onset preeclampsia and its complications.

■ Conclusion

In conclusion, preeclampsia remains a major cause of maternal and fetal morbidity. The substantial loss of life as well as serious long-term sequelae of preeclampsia could be largely eliminated if we could accurately predict, prevent, and better manage the disease. It is evident at the present time that there is no clinically useful test to accurately predict preeclampsia. The tests that seem to offer the promise of both a high positive likelihood ratio and low negative likelihood ratio are the pro- and anti-angiogenic factors (sFlt-1, sEng, PlGF, VEGF), PP-13, and combinations of these serum markers with uterine artery Doppler velocimetry. Further large prospective clinical studies are required to establish the real potential of these markers as individual predictive tests and to identify the ideal combination of tests for combined, sequential, and multiple testing. However, in the absence of any proven preventative strategy or treatment for preeclampsia, women identified as being at high risk of developing this disorder may experience considerable anxiety. Additional studies are needed to evaluate the impact of early diagnosis on overall pregnancy outcome.

REFERENCES

1. Villar J, Say L, Gulmezoglu AM, *et al*. Eclampsia and preeclampsia: a worldwide health problem for 2000 years. In: MacLean A, Poston L, Walker J, eds. *Preeclampsia*. London, RCOG Press. 2003;189–207.
2. Newman RB, Eddy GL. Association of eclampsia and hydatidiform mole: case report and review of the literature. *Obstet Gynecol Surv* 1988;**43**(4):185–90.
3. Roberts JM. Endothelial dysfunction in preeclampsia. *Semin Reprod Endocrinol* 1998;**16**(1):5–15.
4. Conde-Agudelo A, Villar J, Lindheimer M. World Health Organization systematic review of screening tests for preeclampsia. *Obstet Gynecol* 2004;**104**(6): 1367–91.
5. Meekins JW, Pijnenborg R, Hanssens M, McFadyen IR, van Asshe A. A study of placental bed spiral arteries and trophoblast invasion in normal and severe preeclamptic pregnancies. *Br J Obstet Gynaecol* 1994;**101**(8):669–74.
6. Olofsson P, Laurini RN, Marsal K. A high uterine artery pulsatility index reflects a defective development of placental bed spiral arteries in pregnancies complicated by hypertension and fetal growth retardation. *Eur J Obstet Gynecol Reprod Biol* 1993;**49**(3):161–8.

7. Cnossen JS, Morris RK, ter Riet G, *et al.* Use of uterine artery Doppler ultrasonography to predict pre-eclampsia and intrauterine growth restriction: a systematic review and bivariable meta-analysis. *CMAJ* 2008;**178**(6):701–11.

8. Pilalis A, Souka AP, Antsaklis P, *et al.* Screening for pre-eclampsia and fetal growth restriction by uterine artery Doppler and PAPP-A at 11–14 weeks' gestation. *Ultrasound Obstet Gynecol* 2007;**29**(2):135–40.

9. Spencer K, Cowans NJ, Chefetz I, Tal J, Meiri H. First-trimester maternal serum PP-13, PAPP-A and second-trimester uterine artery Doppler pulsatility index as markers of pre-eclampsia. *Ultrasound Obstet Gynecol* 2007;**29**(2):128–34.

10. Crispi F, Llurba E, Dominguez C, *et al.* Predictive value of angiogenic factors and uterine artery Doppler for early-versus late-onset pre-eclampsia and intrauterine growth restriction. *Ultrasound Obstet Gynecol* 2008;**31**(3):303–9.

11. Stepan H, Geipel A, Schwartz F, *et al.* Circulatory soluble endoglin and its predictive value for preeclampsia in second-trimester pregnancies with abnormal uterine perfusion. *Am J Obstet Gynecol* 2008;**198**(2):175.e1–6.

12. Than NG, Pick E, Bellyei S, *et al.* Functional analyses of placental protein 13/galectin-13. *Eur J Biochem* 2004;**271**(6):1065–78.

13. Nicolaides KH, Bindra R, Turan OM, *et al.* A novel approach to first-trimester screening for early pre-eclampsia combining serum PP-13 and Doppler ultrasound. *Ultrasound Obstet Gynecol* 2006;**27**(1):13–17.

14. Chafetz I, Kuhnreich I, Sammar M, *et al.* First-trimester placental protein 13 screening for preeclampsia and intrauterine growth restriction. *Am J Obstet Gynecol* 2007;**197**(1):35.e1–7.

15. Romero R, Kusanoric JP, Than NG, *et al.* First-trimester maternal serum PP13 in the risk assessment for preeclampsia. *Am J Obstet Gynecol* 2008;**199**(2):122.e1–11.

16. Koga K, Osuga Y, Yoshino O, *et al.* Elevated serum soluble vascular endothelial growth factor receptor 1 (sVEGFR-1) levels in women with preeclampsia. *J Clin Endocrinol Metab* 2003;**88**(5):2348–51.

17. Maynard SE, Min JY, Merchan J, *et al.* Excess placental soluble fms-like tyrosine kinase 1 (sFlt1) may contribute to endothelial dysfunction, hypertension, and proteinuria in preeclampsia. *J Clin Invest* 2003;**111**(5):649–58.

18. Levine RJ, Maynard SE, Qian C, *et al.* Circulating angiogenic factors and the risk of preeclampsia. *N Engl J Med* 2004;**350**(7):672–83.

19. McKeeman GC, Ardill JE, Caldwell CM, Hunter AJ, McClure N. Soluble vascular endothelial growth factor receptor-1 (sFlt-1) is increased throughout gestation in patients who have preeclampsia develop. *Am J Obstet Gynecol* 2004;**191**(4):1240–6.

20. Ahmad S, Ahmed A. Elevated placental soluble vascular endothelial growth factor receptor-1 inhibits angiogenesis in preeclampsia. *Circ Res* 2004;**95**(9):884–91.

21. Dvorak HF. Vascular permeability factor/vascular endothelial growth factor: a critical cytokine in tumor angiogenesis and a potential target for diagnosis and therapy. *J Clin Oncol* 2002;**20**(21):4368–80.

22. Ferrara N, Davis-Smyth T. The biology of vascular endothelial growth factor. *Endocr Rev* 1997;**18**(1):4–25.

23. Kendall RL, Wang G, Thomas KA. Identification of a natural soluble form of the vascular endothelial growth factor receptor, FLT-1, and its heterodimerization with KDR. *Biochem Biophys Res Commun* 1996;**226**(2):324–8.

24. Levine RJ, Lam C, Qian C, *et al*. CPEP Study Group Soluble endoglin and other circulating antiangiogenic factors in preeclampsia. *N Engl J Med* 2006;**355** (10):992–1005.

25. Venkatesha S, Torporsian M, Lam C, *et al*. Soluble endoglin contributes to the pathogenesis of preeclampsia. *Nat Med* 2006;**12**(6):642–9.

26. Zhou Y, McMaster M, Woo K, *et al*. Vascular endothelial growth factor ligands and receptors that regulate human cytotrophoblast survival are dysregulated in severe preeclampsia and hemolysis, elevated liver enzymes, and low platelets syndrome. *Am J Pathol* 2002;**160**(4):1405–23.

27. Chaiworapongsa T, Romero R, Espinoza J, *et al*. Evidence supporting a role for blockade of the vascular endothelial growth factor system in the pathophysiology of preeclampsia. Young Investigator Award. *Am J Obstet Gynecol* 2004; **190**(6):1541–7; discussion 1547–50.

28. Shibata E, Rajakumar A, Powers RW, *et al*. Soluble fms-like tyrosine kinase 1 is increased in preeclampsia but not in normotensive pregnancies with small-for-gestational-age neonates: relationship to circulating placental growth factor. *J Clin Endocrinol Metab* 2005;**90**(8):4895–903.

29. Buhimschi CS, Norwitz ER, Funai E, *et al*. Urinary angiogenic factors cluster hypertensive disorders and identify women with severe preeclampsia. *Am J Obstet Gynecol* 2005;**192**(3):734–41.

30. Levine RJ, Thadhani R, Qian C, *et al*. Urinary placental growth factor and risk of preeclampsia. *JAMA* 2005;**293**(1):77–85.

31. Aggarwal PK, Jain V, Sakhuja V, Karumanchi SA, Jha V. Low urinary placental growth factor is a marker of pre-eclampsia. *Kidney Int* 2006;**69**(3):621–4.

32. Signore C, Mills JL, Qian C, *et al*. Circulating angiogenic factors and placental abruption. *Obstet Gynecol* 2006;**108**(2):338–44.

33. Signore C, Mills JL, Qian C, *et al*. Circulating soluble endoglin and placental abruption. *Prenat Diagn* 2008;**28**(9):852–8.

34. Hertig A, Berkane N, Leferre G, *et al*. Maternal serum sFlt1 concentration is an early and reliable predictive marker of preeclampsia. *Clin Chem* 2004;**50**(9): 1702–3.

35. Chaiworapongsa T, Romero R, Kim YM, *et al*. Plasma soluble vascular endothelial growth factor receptor-1 concentration is elevated prior to the clinical diagnosis of pre-eclampsia. *J Matern Fetal Neonatal Med* 2005;**17**(1):3–18.

36. Wathen KA, Tuutti E, Stenman UH, *et al*. Maternal serum-soluble vascular endothelial growth factor receptor-1 in early pregnancy ending in preeclampsia or intrauterine growth retardation. *J Clin Endocrinol Metab* 2006;**91** (1):180–4.

37. Rana S, Karumanchi SA, Levine RJ, *et al.* Sequential changes in antiangiogenic factors in early pregnancy and risk of developing preeclampsia. *Hypertension* 2007;**50**(1):137–42.

38. Vatten LJ, Eskild A, Nilsen TI, *et al.* Changes in circulating level of angiogenic factors from the first to second trimester as predictors of preeclampsia. *Am J Obstet Gynecol* 2007;**196**(3):239.e1–6.

39. Widmer M, Villar J, Benigni A, *et al.* Mapping the theories of preeclampsia and the role of angiogenic factors: a systematic review. *Obstet Gynecol* 2007;**109**(1): 168–80.

40. Thomas CP, Andrews JI, Liu KZ. Intronic polyadenylation signal sequences and alternate splicing generate human soluble Flt1 variants and regulate the abundance of soluble Flt1 in the placenta. *FASEB J* 2007;**21**(14):3885–95.

41. Sela S, Itin A, Natanson-Yaron S, *et al.* A novel human-specific soluble vascular endothelial growth factor receptor 1: cell-type-specific splicing and implications to vascular endothelial growth factor homeostasis and preeclampsia. *Circ Res* 2008;**102**(12):1566–74.

42. Bills VL, Varet J, Millar A, *et al.* Failure to up-regulate VEGF165b in maternal plasma is a first trimester predictive marker for pre-eclampsia. *Clin Sci (Lond)* 2009;**116**(3):265–72.

43. Wallukat G, Homuth V, Fischer T, *et al.* Patients with preeclampsia develop agonistic autoantibodies against the angiotensin AT1 receptor. *J Clin Invest* 1999;**103**(7):945–52.

44. Xia Y, Wen H, Bobst S, Day MC, Kellems RE. Maternal autoantibodies from preeclamptic patients activate angiotensin receptors on human trophoblast cells. *J Soc Gynecol Investig* 2003;**10**(2):82–93.

45. Zhou CC, Zhang Y, Irani RA, *et al.* Angiotensin receptor agonistic autoantibodies induce pre-eclampsia in pregnant mice. *Nat Med* 2008;**14**(8):855–62.

46. Fu ML, Hertitz H, Schulze W, *et al.* Autoantibodies against the angiotensin receptor (AT1) in patients with hypertension. *J Hypertens* 2000;**18**(7):945–53.

47. Karumanchi SA, Lindheimer MD. Preeclampsia pathogenesis: "triple a rating"-autoantibodies and antiangiogenic factors. *Hypertension* 2008;**51**(4):991–2.

48. Speer PD, Powers RW, Frank MP, *et al.* Elevated asymmetric dimethylarginine concentrations precede clinical preeclampsia, but not pregnancies with small-for-gestational-age infants. *Am J Obstet Gynecol* 2008;**198**(1):112.e1–7.

49. Savvidou MD, Hingorani AD, Tsikas D, *et al.* Endothelial dysfunction and raised plasma concentrations of asymmetric dimethylarginine in pregnant women who subsequently develop pre-eclampsia. *Lancet* 2003;**361**(9368):1511–17.

50. Poon LC, Kametas NA, Maiz N, Akolekar R, Nicolaides KH. First-trimester prediction of hypertensive disorders in pregnancy. *Hypertension* 2009;**53**(5): 812–18.

Preexisting hypertension in pregnancy

5

Ellen Knox, Mark Kilby, and Louise C. Kenny

■ Definition

Chronic hypertension complicates 1–2% of pregnancies and its incidence may be underestimated [1]. It is defined as persistent hypertension that presents before pregnancy or within the first 20 weeks of gestation [2].

Women may be identified as being hypertensive in the primary care setting, prior to pregnancy. The rise in maternal age, and the proportion of women with raised body mass index (BMI) $> 30 \, \text{kg/m}^2$ and with insulin resistance, all of which are associated with a significant risk of hypertension, are likely to make this an increasingly common occurrence. In contrast, apparently healthy young women will not have had their blood pressure checked prior to pregnancy and thus chronic hypertension may manifest for the first time at booking. Chronic hypertension (if not identified pre-pregnancy) may be "masked" by physiological hemodynamic changes in pregnancy, in particular the second trimester reduction in arterial blood pressure, secondary to increasing vasodilatation. A prospective review of women who underwent renal biopsies close to pregnancy revealed that a small but significant number of women have underlying preexisting renal disease presenting initially in pregnancy as preeclampsia [3]. Of the 40 women with proteinuria, with or without preeclampsia, that persisted postnatally, 19 had chronic kidney disease stage 3–5 and 6 had end-stage renal failure at follow-up. Therefore, medical and midwifery staff need to be increasingly aware of and prepared for these conditions and to arrange appropriate investigation and follow-up.

5

Hypertension in Pregnancy, ed. Alexander Heazell, Errol R. Norwitz, Louise C. Kenny, and Philip N. Baker. Published by Cambridge University Press. © Cambridge University Press 2010.

Cardiovascular disease accounted for 40% of all deaths among women in the UK in 2002 [4]. Pregnancy may provide a window of opportunity to detect those at high risk and implement potentially lifesaving treatment and lifestyle modifications. Clearly the duty of the obstetrician is to optimize management during pregnancy, which includes timely screening and investigation and advice on pharmacoprophylaxis and antihypertensive treatment in an attempt to reduce maternal and fetal morbidity and mortality. Such an obligation should track into the puerperium where appropriate investigation and treatment may be instituted.

■ Adverse pregnancy outcome

Chronic maternal hypertension is associated with relatively poor pregnancy outcomes [5–7]. A systematic review of the literature relating to the investigation and treatment of mild chronic hypertension in pregnancy has demonstrated a twofold increase risk in placental abruption (odds ratio [OR], 2.1; 95% confidence interval [CI], 1.1–3.9), a threefold increase risk in overall perinatal mortality (OR 3.4, 95% CI, 3.0–3.7), and an increase in proportion of small-for-gestational-age infants, prematurity, and low birthweight [6].

Data from a review of observational studies of women with mild chronic hypertension report the following range of association with adverse pregnancy outcome [7]:

- Superimposed preeclampsia 10–25%
- Placental abruption 0.7–1.5%
- Preterm birth prior to 37 weeks 12–34%
- Fetal growth restriction 8–16%.

These outcomes have a much higher prevalence in women with severe chronic hypertension in the first trimester (preeclampsia 50%, abruption 5–10%, preterm birth 62–70%, growth restriction 31–40%) and are higher still in women with severe hypertension and superimposed preeclampsia.

A retrospective cohort study of obstetric patients with chronic renal disease involving 358 women from the maternity hospitals in Birmingham, Leicester, and Hammersmith in London compared pregnancy outcomes with a control cohort of 113 782 women without renal disease [8]. Chronic hypertension (treated or untreated, with diastolic blood pressures of 90 mmHg or above) was associated with neonatal death and preterm birth. Hypertension was also associated with a reduction in pregnancy duration whatever the severity of renal impairment. Perinatal risk increased in parallel with increased baseline maternal renal dysfunction.

■ Maternal evaluation

The diagnosis of hypertension as defined by blood pressure of $\geq 140/90$ mmHg prior to or during the early part of pregnancy should prompt investigation for associated disease processes such as diabetes, and secondary causes such as renal, cardiac, or collagen vascular disease and assessment of end-organ damage. A full personal and family history should in particular enquire about history of recurrent urinary tract infections, photosensitive skin lesions, and arthropathy. Clinical examination at presentation should include palpation of femoral pulses (to elicit or exclude radiofemoral delay).

The following investigations should be performed:
- Urinalysis (evaluation of proteinuria and the exclusion of red cell casts)
- Urinary dipstick analysis alone is inaccurate in determining significant (> 0.3 g protein/24 hours) proteinuria but a finding of 1+ or more should prompt quantification [9]. A recent systematic review of 13 studies found the spot protein:creatinine ratio < 30 mg/mmol to be a reasonable alternative to exclude significant proteinuria [10]. Within this review two studies examined the albumin:creatinine ratio and this was found to have good correlation with a diagnosis of > 0.3 g protein on 24-hour analysis. Currently, analysis of 24-hour urine protein collection remains the most extensively studied and further studies examining spot tests (e.g., protein:creatinine ratio) and correlation with adverse pregnancy outcomes are required.
- Midstream urine (to exclude occult urinary tract infection by microscopy, culture, and sensitivity)
- Serum urea, creatinine, and electrolytes: to define baseline maternal renal biochemistry and screen for hypokalemia in Conn's syndrome.
- Electrocardiogram (ECG) in cases of chronic hypertension to exclude left ventricular hypertrophy. In specific cases it may be necessary to obtain an echocardiogram.
- Renal ultrasound scan to exclude congenital renal tract anomalies, screen for adult polycystic renal disease, and renal parenchymal scarring.

- Very rarely, intractable, "brittle" and severe hypertension may lead the clinician to consider the diagnosis of a pheochromocytoma. Additional symptoms of sweating, headache, and palpitations may heighten suspicion of this diagnosis further. Fetal and maternal mortality is high in undiagnosed cases and labor may precipitate a hypertensive crisis. A 24-hour urine save should be sent for urinary vanillylmandelic acid or catecholamines (both of which are raised) if this is suspected.

- Consideration should also be given to checking for maternal anticardiolipin antibodies and circulating lupus anticoagulant based on previous obstetric and personal history (i.e., co-existent pregnancies losses, previous severe early-onset preeclampsia, or arterial/venous thromboembolic disease).

■ Pre-pregnancy

In those cases of known preexisting hypertension, evaluation should begin preconceptually. The above secondary causes and associations should be excluded if not previously investigated. Pre-pregnancy management should involve a review of antihypertensive control. It is estimated that only a quarter of patients with known hypertension are adequately treated. A review of patients with chronic kidney disease indicates that treatment is no better and may be worse [11]. This is of concern as suboptimal treatment will propagate worsening kidney function by direct antihypertensive effect on the nephrons and an increase in cardiovascular morbidity and mortality. The importance of good control should be emphasized to those embarking on a pregnancy.

In the pre-pregnancy consultation there should be a review of antihypertensive medication. In the non-pregnant population with chronic kidney disease, it is important to manage both components of hypertension – vasoconstriction and hypervolemia. Therefore, antihypertensive therapy often involves a renin–angiotensin–aldosterone blocker which largely eliminates vasoconstriction and some of the sympathetic over activity [12]. Long-term outcome studies treating chronic kidney disease using angiotensin converting enzyme (ACE) inhibitors or angiotensinogen II receptor blockers (ARBs) show long-term improvement in renal function. This is most beneficial if protein excretion is $< 1\,g/day$, but improved renal outcome occurs even in the presence of more severe proteinuria [13]. However, renin–angiotensin–aldosterone blockers are contraindicated in pregnancy because of their association with fetal growth restriction, perinatal renal failure, and probably cardiac and neurological congenital abnormalities [14]. Therefore, they should ideally be discontinued pre-pregnancy and replaced by one of the therapeutic agents with an improved safety profile in pregnancy.

Women with mild to moderate uncomplicated chronic hypertension may be able to stop their antihypertensives at the booking visit in the presence of normotension and careful monitoring. Antihypertensives may be discontinued in the second trimester as a result of the normal reduction of blood pressure at this time. Target values for treatment depend upon the underlying pathology as discussed below and there remains some controversy regarding the optimal blood pressure for maternal and fetal well-being.

■ Aims of treatment

- There is no evidence that treatment prevents the adverse pregnancy conditions of superimposed preeclampsia and abruption or improves fetal or maternal outcome [15–19], with the exception of a reduction in the development of severe hypertension later in pregnancy [18–20].
- There are benefits for the reduction of blood pressure values to < 160 mmHg systolic and < 110 mmHg diastolic, above which there is a strong risk of stroke. In addition, maternal morbidity such as renal failure and heart failure in secondary hypertension is potentially improved.
- The mean arterial blood pressure (MAP) in the first and second trimester is a better predictor of subsequent preeclampsia than systolic blood pressure, diastolic blood pressure, or an increase in blood pressure [21].
- Ambulatory blood pressure readings in pregnancy potentially avoid "white coat" hypertension and demonstrate the diurnal variation in blood pressure which is not present in preeclampsia [22]. Normal pregnancy values have been evaluated. Ambulatory blood pressure has a better correlation with hypertensive complications of pregnancy [23].

Mild to moderate hypertension

There is currently insufficient evidence to support the treatment of mild to moderate hypertension (systolic 140–169 mmHg/diastolic 90–109 mmHg) in pregnancy. A Cochrane review of 46 trials (4289 women) did show a reduction of severe hypertension but no improvement in the development of preeclampsia, preterm birth, small-for-gestational-age infants, or fetal death [24].

Currently a randomized controlled trial (Control of Hypertension in Pregnancy Study [CHIPS]) is underway to determine whether tight versus less tight control of mild to moderate hypertension improves pregnancy outcome. The initial pilot study involved women in 17 obstetric centers in the UK, Canada, Australia, and New Zealand [25]. The entry criteria were: preexisting/gestational hypertension, diastolic blood pressure 90–109 mmHg, live fetus(es), and duration of pregnancy 20 weeks to 33 weeks and 6 days. Subjects were randomized to less tight (target diastolic blood pressure 100 mmHg) versus tight (target diastolic blood pressure 85 mmHg) control. One hundred and thirty-two women were randomized in total, 66 to less tight (7 excluded as no study visit) and 66 to tight (one lost to follow up and 7 had no study visit). Tight control resulted in a significant lowering of mean diastolic blood pressure (–3.5 mmHg, 95% CI –6.4 to –0.6). With less tight (versus tight) control, the rates of other treatments and outcomes were as follows:

- Post-randomization antenatal antihypertensive medication use 46 (69.7%) versus 58 (89.2%)
- Severe hypertension 38 (57.6%) versus 26 (40%)
- Proteinuria 16 (24.2%) versus 20 (30.8%)
- Serious maternal complications 3 (4.6%) versus 2 (3.1%)
- Preterm birth 24 (36.4%) versus 26 (40%)
- Birthweight 2675 + 858 g versus 2501 + 855 g
- Neonatal intensive care unit admission 15 (22.7%) versus 22 (34.4%)
- Serious perinatal complications 9 (13.6%) versus 14 (21.5%).

Compliance in both groups was 79% and maternal satisfaction was good [26]. The ongoing substantive trial will be sufficiently powered to examine outcomes such as perinatal loss.

Complicated and secondary hypertension

Those women that have underlying reasons or associations with their mild to moderate hypertension may benefit from treatment to reduce maternal sequelae. These groups include [7,17]:

- Secondary hypertension (renal disease, coarctation of the aorta, collagen vascular disease)
- End-organ damage
- Dyslipidemia

- Microvascular disease
- History of stroke
- Diabetes
- Maternal age over 40.

Target values for treatment in these groups have been suggested at levels below 140/90 mmHg. In non-pregnant patients with chronic renal failure and hypertension, the target blood pressure is 130/80 mmHg according to the seventh Report of the Joint National Committee in the USA [27]. Two multicenter outcome studies led to this conclusion, showing improved cardiovascular outcome in patients with microvascular disease and renal disease with lower levels of blood pressure [28,29]. However, the value of targets this low in pregnancy has not been established.

Severe hypertension

Severe hypertension (blood pressure > 160 mmHg systolic or diastolic > 110 mmHg) should be treated to minimize maternal conditions of stroke, renal failure, and heart failure. Care should be given to avoid precipitous drops in arterial blood pressure, which may be detrimental both to the mother and feto-placental perfusion. This warrants inpatient monitoring and may require intravenous therapy with labetalol or hydralazine. In these situations monitoring with an arterial line and titration of the dose to response in blood pressure is required.

■ Which antihypertensive to use?

There is a dearth of large well-designed randomized controlled trials on which to base treatment recommendations on. All drugs used cross the placenta.

As previously mentioned, ACE inhibitors and ARBs should not be used in pregnancy and should ideally be discontinued pre-pregnancy (see pre-pregnancy counseling).

Currently either methyldopa or labetalol are recommended as first-line agents, with the addition of a long-acting calcium channel blocker such as nifedipine as a second or third therapy.

First-line drugs

Methyldopa is the preferred drug of the National High Blood Pressure Education Program for pregnancy [30]. It is a centrally acting drug, and has the longest follow-up of childhood data following in utero exposure [18,31]. It does not alter uteroplacental or fetal dynamics. However, it is a mild antihypertensive and many women fail to gain blood pressure control on this drug alone [19,31]. In addition, many find the side effect of sedation troublesome.

Labetalol has less maternal side effects than methyldopa and is the most extensively used beta-adrenergic blocker in pregnancy. It is not selective and has some alpha-adrenergic blockade. Labetalol may preserve uteroplacental blood flow more than beta-adrenergic blockers such as atenolol that have been associated with lower placental and fetal weight at delivery when started early in pregnancy [32–35]. Propranolol, which is a non-selective beta-adrenergic blocker, has been associated with fetal growth restriction, bradycardia, and hypoglycemia as well as preterm labor and neonatal apnoea [36]. This may be related to counteracting the β_2-receptor-mediated myometrial relaxation. A systematic review comparing beta-blockers with methyldopa showed them to be better at reducing severe hypertension [16]. Beta-blockers should not be given to women with asthma. A review of beta-blockers showed a reduction in severe hypertension (risk ratio [RR], 0.37; 95%, CI 0.26–0.53) and a reduction in the need for additional hypertensives (RR, 0.44; 95% CI, 0.31–0.62) [24]. There were insufficient data for perinatal mortality or prematurity to be examined. There was an increased association with small for gestational age (RR, 1.36; 95% CI, 1.02–1.82). Thirteen trials of 854 women compared methyldopa to beta-blockers and showed them to be no more effective and equally as safe.

Second-line agents

Calcium-channel blockers such as long-acting nifedipine appear safe in pregnancy despite earlier concerns that they may affect uteroplacental blood flow [18,36]. Maternal side effects include headache and facial flushing. Sublingual therapy should not be given because of the precipitous drop in blood pressure which may be particularly harmful to the uteroplacental unit. Outside of pregnancy, there is experience with amlodipine but this is lacking in pregnancy.

Thiazide diuretic therapy is controversial because of the risk of volume depletion. However, in chronic usage this is unlikely as all of the fluid loss occurs during the first two weeks of therapy as long as drug dose and dietary sodium remain constant. Current recommendations are that they can be continued as long as volume depletion is avoided [31,37].

■ Place of treatment

- There is evidence from one small trial that non-proteinuric hypertension can be managed as an outpatient in day assessment units, thereby reducing hospital inpatient stay [38].
- Secondary hypertension is best managed in joint clinics with obstetricians and physicians with experience in the underlying condition.

■ Prevention of superimposed preeclampsia in at-risk patients

The treatment of chronic hypertension in pregnancy has not been shown to reduce the incidence of preeclampsia. However, much work has been done researching other potential prophylactic agents, which are discussed below.

- Consideration should be given to commencing low-dose aspirin. Large randomized controlled trials failed to demonstrate a benefit to the general pregnant population but provided reassuring safety data for its usage [39,40]. Subsequent studies have shown a reduction in superimposed preeclampsia in women at increased risk, although this has not been a universal finding. The most recent meta-analysis of individual patient data from the PARIS group examined 32 217 women in 31 randomized controlled trials and concluded that the number needed to treat to reduce one case of preeclampsia is 50 [41]. In addition to a reduction in preeclampsia (RR, 0.9; 95% CI, 0.84–0.97) there was a reduction in delivery before 34 weeks (RR, 0.9; 95% CI, 0.83–0.98) and a reduction in pregnancies with a serious adverse outcome (RR, 0.9; 95% CI, 0.85–0.96).
- There has been interest in the use of antioxidant medication in pregnancy. However, critical appraisal of the literature has indicated that there is no place for the use of oral vitamin C or E in pharmacoprophylaxis. Following the in vitro evidence of uteroplacental and systemic oxidative stress in preeclampsia, it was hypothesized that antioxidants may reduce preeclampsia in high-risk groups. This was addressed by the Vitamins in Pregnancy (VIP) study a randomized controlled trial in which 2404 women were randomized to receive

antioxidants vitamin C and E (n = 1199) or matched placebo (n = 1205). Those women receiving the vitamins E and C had a non-significant decrease in preeclampsia (RR 0.97 95% CI 0.8–1.17), more severe hypertension, lower birthweight babies and increased perinatal morbidity (risk of stillbirth < 24 weeks 2.70; 95% CI, 1.02–7.14) [42].

- Calcium supplementation with at least 1 g calcium daily reduces the risk of preeclampsia by between 31% and 67% [43]. The effect is most marked for those with reduced calcium intake and those at high risk. An inverse relationship between calcium intake and subsequent preeclampsia was first described in 1980 and led to the hypothesis that calcium supplementation may reduce risk of subsequent preeclampsia [44]. The World Health Organization trial of calcium supplementation randomized 8325 nulliparous normotensive women with low dietary calcium intake to placebo versus 1.5 g calcium daily prior to 20 weeks. Although this failed to show a reduction in preeclampsia incidence, those developing the disease did so at a later gestation, had a lower incidence of eclampsia (RR, 0.68; 95% CI, 0.48–0.97) and severe hypertensive complications (RR, 0.71; 95% CI, 0.61–0.82) and had a lower perinatal morbidity (RR, 0.7; 95% CI, 0.56–0.88) [45].

■ Fetal assessment

- First-trimester ultrasound has been shown to accurately date pregnancies and this is important particularly when delivery may be premature and avoids uncertainty regarding gestation if a later scan reveals a small fetus.
- Uterine artery Dopplers at 24 weeks have been shown to be associated with the development of preeclampsia in a high-risk group [46]. The most recent review of 74 studies of 79 547 women revealed that an increased pulsatility index with notching in the second trimester best predicted overall preeclampsia (positive likelihood ratio 21.0 among high-risk patients) [47].
- In the presence of co-existent preeclampsia or growth restriction, close fetal surveillance with serial growth scans and additional tests of fetal well-being such as umbilical artery Doppler (e.g., middle cerebral artery, Ductus Venosus) should be performed. Supplementary Doppler

studies may be required at the extremes of gestation and in the presence of severe growth restriction to aid delivery timing.

- In the absence of preeclampsia or growth restriction, the frequency of fetal surveillance and its need are controversial. However, there is evidence from a meta-analysis that a reduction in MAP induced by antihypertensive treatment affects fetal growth [48]. A decrease in MAP of 10 mmHg was associated with a 176 g fall in birthweight, independent of the type of hypertension or drug therapy used. This and evidence from the CHIPS pilot which showed a lower birthweight following very tight blood pressure control would appear to support the rationale of fetal surveillance, at least involving serial growth, liquor volume, and umbilical artery Doppler scans for women whose hypertension is being treated [25].
- Suppressed fetal growth in utero is now thought to have long-term detrimental health consequences. Evidence surrounding the Barker hypothesis suggests that fetal undernutrition confers later risk of cardiovascular disease [49]. This therefore potentially identifies a cohort of individuals who may benefit from lifestyle interventions and close surveillance.

■ Special considerations for labor and delivery

- The timing of delivery will depend upon the presence of superimposed preeclampsia and any other evidence of maternal or fetal compromise.
- In the presence of well-controlled uncomplicated hypertension induction of labor may be delayed until 40 weeks' gestation.
- Ergometrine should not be given to women with hypertension for the third stage or treatment of postpartum hemorrhage because of the risk of precipitous rises in blood pressure.

■ Postnatal assessment

- Postnatal management should involve optimizing blood pressure control without the fear of reducing blood pressure too low for the potential detriment of the feto-placental unit.
- Superimposed preeclampsia may still occur postnatally and women should be warned to report symptoms of headache, visual disturbances, and epigastric pain and receive prompt assessment if these occur.

Eclampsia has been recorded as late as four weeks postnatally. However, the principle risk time is the first four days and women with severe preeclampsia or eclampsia should stay in for at least this length of time.

- In the absence of preeclampsia the presence of uncomplicated mild to moderate hypertension should not delay discharge although anti-hypertensives should not be discontinued immediately prior to home.

- Clear instructions should be given prior to discharge regarding the frequency of midwifery review of blood pressure and acceptable target blood pressures that warrant review. These will depend upon the underlying cause and severity of hypertension. In addition the need for general practice review of medication should be communicated.

- Post-pregnancy hospital review should be offered for those with pregnancy complications and appropriate multidisciplinary review for those with secondary hypertension.

- Post-pregnancy management may involve recommencing ACE inhibitors and appropriate follow-up to minimize long-term sequelae of hypertension, as well as instruction on the importance of pre-pregnancy assessment prior to subsequent pregnancies.

- In view of the aforementioned increased cardiovascular risks following gestational hypertension and preeclampsia, the British Hypertension Society recommends regular blood pressure monitoring for those women post-pregnancy. However, they do not state the frequency of that assessment. After normotension has been achieved it would seem reasonable to monitor blood pressure at least on an annual basis. In addition lifestyle modifications such as diet and exercise, stopping smoking, and modification of alcohol intake should be discussed.

- Venous thromboembolism remains the leading cause of maternal mortality in the UK and all women should be assessed for their risk and need for prophylaxis with thromboembolic stockings and heparin. Women with hypertension, particularly with superimposed preeclampsia, may be at increased risk especially with the potential co-existence of obesity and immobility.

■ Conclusion

Chronic hypertension may be detected for the first time in pregnancy. It is important that it is fully investigated and managed appropriately, with the aim of optimizing pregnancy outcome and influencing future maternal health.

REFERENCES

1. Roberts CL, Bell JC, Ford JB, *et al.* The accuracy of reporting of the hypertensive disorders of pregnancy in population health data. *Hypertens Pregnancy* 2008;**27**:285–97.

2. Brown MA, Lindheimer MD, DeSwiet M, *et al.* The classification and diagnosis of the hypertensive disorders of pregnancy: statement from the International Society of the Study of Hypertension in Pregnancy. *Hypertens Pregnancy* 2001;**20**:IX–XIV.

3. Day C, Hewins P, Hildebrabd S, *et al.* The role of renal biopsy in women with kidney disease identified in pregnancy. *Nephrol Dial Transplant* 2008;**23**:201–6.

4. World Health OrganiSation. Numbers and Rates of Registered Deaths, United Kingdom 2002. www.who.int/whosis/database/mort/table1_process. cmf#demographic.

5. Rey E, Couturier A. The prognosis of pregnancy in women with chronic hypertension. *Am J Obstet Gynecol* 1994;**171**:410–16.

6. Ferrier RL, Sibai BM, Mulrow CD, *et al.* Management of mild chronic hypertension during pregnancy: a review. *Obstet Gynecol* 2000;**96**:849–60.

7. Sibai BM, Lindheimer MD, Hauth J, *et al.* Risk factors for pre-eclampsia, abruption placentae, and adverse neonatal outcome amongst women with chronic hypertension. *N Engl J Med* 1998;**339**:667–71.

8. Ferraro A, Somerset DA, Lipkin G, *et al.* Pregnancy in women with pre-existing renal diease: maternal and fetal outcomes. *J Obstet Gynaecol* 2005;**25**:S13.

9. Waugh JJ, Clark TJ, Divakaran TG, Khan KS, Kilby MD. Accuracy of urinalysis dipstick techniques in predicting significant proteinuria in pregnancy. *Obstet Gynecol* 2004;**103**:769–77.

10. Cote AM, Brown MA, Lam E, *et al.* Diagnostic accuracy of urinary spot protein: creatinine ratio for protein in hypertensive pregnant women: a systematic review. *BMJ* 2008;**336**:1003–6.

11. Schwenger V, Ritz E. Audit of antihypertensive treatment in patients with renal failure. *Nephrol Dial Transplant* 1998;**13**(12):3091–5.

12. Ligtenberg G, Blankestijn PJ, Oey PL, *et al.* Reduction in sympathic overactivity by enalapril in patients with chronic renal failure. *N Engl J Med* 1999;**340**:1321–8.

13. Jafar TH, Stark PC, Schmid CH, *et al.* Progression of chronic renal disease: the role of blood pressure control, proteinuria and angiotensin-converting enzyme inhibition. A patient level meta-analysis. *Ann Intern Med* 2003; **139**:244–52.

14. Sibai BM, Mabie WC, Shamsa F, *et al.* A comparison of no medication versus methyldopa or labetolol in chronic hypertension during pregnancy. *Am J Obstet Gynecol* 1990;**162**:960–6.

15. Remuzzi G, Ruggenenti P. Prevention and treatment of pregnancy-associated hypertension: what have we learned in the last 10 years? *Am J Kidney Dis* 1991;**18**:285.

16. Magee LA, Ornstein MP, von Dadelszen P. Fortnightly review: management of hypertension in pregnancy. *BMJ* 1999;**318**:1332.

17. Abalos E, Duley L, Steyn DW, Henderson-Smart DJ. Antihypertensive drug therapy for mild to moderate hypertension during pregnancy (Cochrane Review). *Cochrane Database Syst Rev* 2001;(2):CD002252.

18. Sibai BM. Chronic hypertension in pregnancy. *Obstet Gynecol* 2002;**100**:369–77.

19. Redman CW. Controlled trials of antihypertensive drugs in pregnancy. *Am J Kidney Dis* 1991;**17**:149–53.

20. National Institutes of Health. *Working Group Report on High Blood Pressure in Pregnancy.* Washington, DC, National Institutes of Health, 2000.

21. Cnossen JS, Vollebregt KC, de Vrieze N, *et al.* Accuracy of mean arterial pressure and blood pressure measurements in predicting pre-eclampsia: systematic review and meta-analysis. *BMJ* 2008;**336**:1117–20.

22. Higgins JR, de Swiet M. Blood-pressure measurement and classification in pregnancy. *Lancet* 2001;**357**(9250):131–5.

23. O'Brien E, Beevers G, Lip GY. ABC of hypertension. Blood pressure measurement. Part III-automated sphygmomanometry: ambulatory blood pressure measurement. *BMJ* 2001;**322**(7294):1110–14.

24. Cochrane Abalos E, Duley L, Steyn DW, Henderson-Smart DJ. Antihypertensive drug therapy for mild to moderate hypertension during pregnancy. *Cochrane Database Syst Rev* 2007;(1):CD002252.

25. Magee LA, von Dadelszen P, Chan S, *et al.* CHIPS Pilot Trial Collaborative Group. The Control of Hypertension In Pregnancy Study pilot trial. *BJOG* 2007;**114**(6):770, e13–20.

26. Magee LA, von Dadelszen P, Chan S, *et al.* Group FT.Women's views of their experiences in the CHIPs (Control of Hypertension in Pregnancy Study) Pilot Trial. *Hypertens Pregnancy.* 2007;**26**(4):371–87.

27. Chobanian AV, Bakris GL, Black HR, *et al.* Seventh Report of the Joint National Committee on Prevention, Detection, Evaluation and Treatment of High Blood Pressure. *Hypertension* 2003;**42**(6):1206–52.

28. Hansson L, Zanchetti A, Carruthers SG, *et al.* Effects of intensive blood-pressure lowering and low-dose aspirin in patients with hypertension: principle results of the Hypertension Optimal Treatment (HOT) randomised trial. HOT Study Group. *Lancet* 1998;**351**:1755–62.

29. Tight blood pressure control and risk of macro- and microvascular complications in type 2 diabetes. UKPDS38. The UK Prospective Diabetes Study Group. *BMJ* 1998;**317**:703–13.

30. NHBPEP. *Report of the National High Blood Pressure Education Project (NJHBPBP) Working Group on High Blood Pressure in Pregnancy.* Washington, DC, National Institutes of Health, NIH publication No 00–3029, July 2000.

31. Ferris TF. Hypertension in pregnancy. *Kidney* 1990;**23**:1.

32. Pickles CJ, Symonds EM, Broughton Pipkin F. The fetal outcome in a randomized double-blind controlled trial of labetalol versus placebo in pregnancy-induced hypertension. *Br J Obstet Gynaecol* 1989;**96**(1):38–43.

33. Montan S, Ingemarsson I, Marsal K, Sjoberg N. Randomised controlled trial of atenolol and pindolol in human pregnancy: effects on fetal hemodynamics. *BMJ* 1992;**304**:946–8.

34. Butters L, Kennedy S, Rubin PC. Atenolol in essential hypertension during pregnancy. *BMJ* 1990;**301**:587–9.

35. Lydakis C, Lip GY, Beevers M, Beevers DG. Atenolol and fetal growth in pregnancies complicated by hypertension. *Am J Hypertens* 1999;**12**:541–7.

36. Magee LA, Duley L. Oral beta-blockers for mild to moderate hypertension during pregnancy. *Cochrane Database Syst Rev* 2003;(3):CD002863.

37. Collins R, Yusuf S, Peto R. Overview of randomised controlled trials of diuretics in pregnancy. *BMJ* 1985;**290**:17–19.

38. Kröner C, Turnbull D, Wilkinson C. Antenatal day care units versus hospital admission for women with complicated pregnancy. *Cochrane Database Syst Rev* 2001;(4):CD001803.

39. Sibai BM, Cartis SN, Thom E, *et al.* Prevention of pre-eclampsia in healthy, nulliparous pregnant women. *N Engl J Med* 1993;**329**:1213–18.

40. CLASP: a randomised trial of low dose aspirin for the prevention and treatment of pre-eclampsia amongst 9364 pregnant women. CLASP (Collaborative Low-dose Aspirin Study in Pregnancy) Collaborative Group *Lancet* 1994;**343**:619–29.

41. Askie LM, Duley L, Henderson-Smart DJ, Stewart LA. PARIS Collaborative Group. *Lancet* 2007;**369**:1765–6.

42. Poston L, Briley A, Seed P, Kelly FJ, Shennan AH. For the VIP trial consortium. Vitamin C and vitamin E in pregnant women at risk for pre-eclampsia: randomised placebo-controlled trial. *Lancet* 2006;**367**:1145–54.

43. Hofmeyer GJ, Atallah AN, Duley L. Calcium supplementation during pregnancy for preventing hypertensive disorders and related problems. *Cochrane Database Syst Rev* 2006;(3):CD001059.

44. Belizan JM, Villar J. The relationship between calcium intake and edema, proteinuria, and hypertension-gestosis: an hypothesis. *Am J Clin Nutr* 1980;**33**:2202–10.

45. Villar J, Abdel-Aleem H, Merialdi M, *et al.* WHO randomised controlled trial of calcium supplementation amongst low calcium intake pregnant women. *Am J Obstet Gynecol* 2006;**194**:639–49.

46. Coleman MA, McCowan LM, North RA. Mid trimester uterine artery Doppler screening as a predictor of adverse pregnancy outcome in high-risk women. *Ultrasound Obstet Gynecol* 2000;**15**(1):7–12.

47. Cnossen JS, Morris RK, ter Riet G, *et al.* Use of uterine artery Doppler ultrasonography to predict pre-eclampsia and intrauterine growth restriction: a systematic review and meta-analysis. *CMAJ* 2008;**178**:701–11.

48. von Dadelszen P, Ornstein MP, Bull SB, *et al.* Fall in mean arterial pressure and fetal growth restriction in pregnancy hypertension: a meta-analysis. *Lancet* 2000;**355**(9198):87–92.

49. Barker DJP. Fetal origins of coronary heart disease. *BMJ* 1995;**311**:171–4.

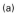

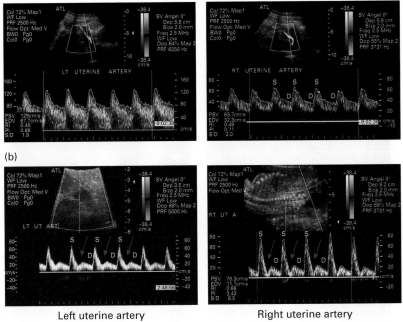

Left uterine artery   Right uterine artery

Figure 4.2 (a) Uterine artery Doppler blood flow in normal pregnancy demonstrating no diastolic notch. (b) Uterine artery notching in a case of preeclampsia (marked with arrows).

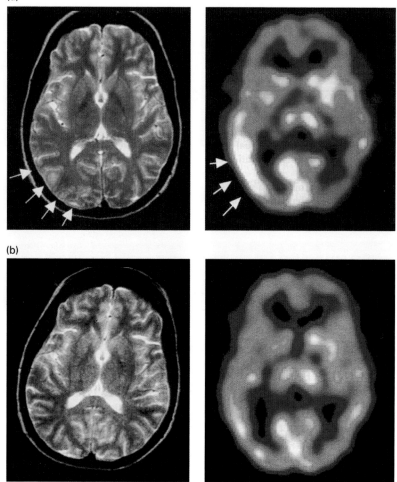

Figure 10.1 Representative head imaging studies of a woman with severe preeclampsia before and after delivery. (a) A representative axial T_2-weighted MRI image (3000 ms/80 ms, TR/TE) of a young woman with severe preeclampsia is shown demonstrating increased T_2 signal (*arrows*) in the peripheral subcortical white matter in the right occipital lobe consistent with hypertensive encephalopathy (left image). A simultaneous axial Tc-99m HMPAO single-photon emission computed tomography image shows increased cerebral perfusion (*arrows*) suggestive of hyperemia in the right posterior temporal cortex, right lateral occipital cortex, and inferior parietal cortex (right image). (b) Follow-up neuroimaging of the same patient eight days after delivery shows marked resolution of both T_2-bright signal on MRI image and of regional hyperperfusion on single-photon emission computed tomography image.

Management of isolated hypertension in pregnancy

6

Arun Jeyabalan and Alexander Heazell

■ Definitions

Gestational hypertension (GH), also referred to as non-proteinuric pregnancy-induced hypertension, is defined by systolic blood pressure ≥ 140 mmHg and/or diastolic blood pressure ≥ 90 mmHg after 20 weeks' gestation in a previously normotensive woman. High blood pressure readings should be sustained with documented elevations on at least two occasions 6 hours apart. Gestational hypertension is classified as severe when blood pressures are consistently greater than 160/110 mmHg, in the absence of proteinuria or other end-organ involvement. The terminology varies geographically in that "gestational hypertension" is used more commonly in the United States [1] whereas "non-proteinuric pregnancy-induced hypertension" is the preferred term in the United Kingdom and Europe [2]. For consistency, GH will be used for the remainder of this chapter.

Gestational hypertension is a provisional diagnosis given during pregnancy and includes women in three major categories: (1) women who will progress to develop preeclampsia, (2) women with "transient hypertension of pregnancy" who do not develop preeclampsia and revert to normal blood pressures by 12 weeks post-delivery, and (3) women that may have previously unrecognized chronic hypertension (high blood pressure first noted after 20 weeks' gestation and persistent elevated blood pressures 12 weeks postpartum). Definitive diagnosis is possible only after reassessment at 6 to 12 weeks postpartum.

Hypertension in Pregnancy, ed. Alexander Heazell, Errol R. Norwitz, Louise C. Kenny, and Philip N. Baker. Published by Cambridge University Press. © Cambridge University Press 2010.

■ Natural history and outcome

The incidence of GH ranges between 6% and 17% among nulliparous women and between 2% and 4% among multiparous women [3–5]. The incidence is higher among women with multiple gestation [6,7]. Although GH and preeclampsia share clinical features, there is controversy whether these represent two distinct pathophysiological entities or rather part of a continuum of the same process. It is estimated that preeclampsia develops in 15–25% of women initially given the diagnosis of GH [8,9]. This is higher than the rate in an unselected obstetric population. The risk of progression to preeclampsia is also inversely proportional to the gestational age at diagnosis of GH, i.e., the earlier the gestational age at which blood pressures are elevated, the higher the risk of developing preeclampsia [8,9]. Barton and colleagues, for example, have reported a 50% rate of progression to preeclampsia among women diagnosed with GH prior to 32 weeks' gestation [8]. Another study reported progression of preeclampsia in 42% of women diagnosed with GH prior to 30 weeks' and 10% among women diagnosed after 36 weeks' gestation [9]. In the HYPITAT trial, a randomized controlled study of labor induction versus expectant management for GH or mild preeclampsia after 36 weeks', progression to severe disease occurred in 36% of expectantly managed subjects and 23% of the women who were induced. However, the rate of progression was not reported separately for the GH group [10].

The precise relationship between perinatal outcomes and GH is also complicated by the limited data for GH as a distinct entity. Outcomes for women with mild GH are generally favorable [5,8,11,12], with rates of preterm birth prior to 37 weeks' ranging from 5% to 17%, preterm birth prior to 34 weeks' 1% to 5%, and fetal growth restriction (FGR) 2% to 14%. Rates of placental abruption and perinatal death with mild GH are also low and estimated to be less than 1%. Earlier studies have also demonstrated no significant effect of GH on perinatal mortality provided that diastolic blood pressure remained less than 110 mmHg [13]. Higher birthweights and later gestational age at delivery have also been reported with mild GH compared with normotensive women [5,11]. Labor induction and Cesarean sections were more common in a cohort of healthy, nulliparous women who developed GH compared with normotensive women [5]. These outcomes were more frequent in women with comorbidities such as gestational diabetes mellitus [14]. The HYPITAT trial which combined GH and mild preeclampsia after 36 weeks' demonstrated a reduced composite adverse maternal outcome of 31% in women who were induced compared with 44% in women who were expectantly managed, with comparable neonatal adverse outcome rates of 6–8% [10].

In contrast, pregnancies complicated by *severe* GH are at increased risk of adverse outcomes at levels comparable with that of severe preeclamspia [11,12]. Buchbinder and colleagues compared perinatal outcomes in women with severe GH to mild preeclampsia and observed higher rates of preterm delivery < 35 weeks' (25% vs. 8.4%) and higher rates of small-for-gestational-age infants (20.8% vs. 6.5%) in the severe GH group. The incidence of placental abruption was comparable with women with severe preeclampsia [12]. The higher incidence of adverse pregnancy outcomes in women with severe GH suggests that this process may be more comparable with severe preeclampsia and therefore possibly different from mild GH.

- Mild GH has minimal effect on perinatal morbidity and mortality.

■ Etiology and pathogenesis

The precise etiology and pathogenesis of hypertensive disorders of pregnancy are not well understood. Not surprisingly, however, GH and preeclampsia appear to share similar pathogenic features. There is evidence of incomplete transformation of uteroplacental spiral arteries [15] and evidence of placental damage including placental infarction in both conditions, but absent intervillous fibrin deposition with GH [16]. In common with placental tissue from preeclampsia, there is also preliminary evidence of dysregulated cell death at the maternal–fetal interface [17]. Interestingly, women with low-lying placenta have a reduced risk of developing GH [18,19]. It has been hypothesized that low-lying placentas have a better developed maternal blood supply, linking GH with placental perfusion and consequent oxidative stress within the placenta.

Gestational hypertension is also associated with an increase in the generation of reactive oxygen species by xanthine oxidase, which is linked to lipid peroxidation and production of hydrogen peroxide [20]. In addition to placental changes, a recent study involving renal biopsy during pregnancy demonstrated glomerular endotheliosis, a lesion thought to be pathognomonic of preeclampsia, in normal pregnancies and pregnancies complicated by GH [21]. It is important to recognize, however, that GH also differs from preeclampsia in several ways; for example, primiparity is a strong risk factor for preeclampsia but not GH, suggesting that the maternal immune dysregulation present in preeclampsia may not be a feature of GH [22].

Gestational hypertension shares some pathological characteristics with preeclampsia. It is also associated with alterations in the concentration of vasoactive factors in the maternal circulation similar to those observed with preeclampsia. While few studies have investigated the concentrations of circulating factors in well-defined subgroups of women with GH, some studies have included women with GH as part of a broader study of women with hypertensive disorders of pregnancy. One such study demonstrated increased levels of endothelin-1, atrial naturetic peptide (ANP), and aldosterone with decreased plasma renin activity [23]. Angiotensin converting enzyme (ACE) activity is also increased in GH [24]. In addition, polymorphisms of the angiotensin-receptor 1 gene are associated with the development of GH perhaps through altered vasoconstrictive actions of angiotensin II [25]. Eicosanoids (prostaglandins and leukotrienes) are also altered in GH, with a decrease in vasodilatory prostaglandins and increase in vasoconstrictive thromboxanes (reviewed by Meagher and FitzGerald [26]).

- Vasoactive circulating factors are altered in GH.

■ Initial evaluation

Major goals in the initial evaluation of pregnant women with elevated blood pressure are to: (1) distinguish between preeclampsia and GH and (2) differentiate between severe and mild hypertensive disorders. These distinctions are important as adverse pregnancy outcomes are higher with preeclampsia and severe GH.

Confirmation of sustained elevated blood pressures and quantification of urinary protein excretion, ideally with a 24-hour timed urine collection, should be a part of the initial evaluation. Symptoms and signs of maternal end-organ damage should also be assessed. This may include questioning the patient regarding symptoms of headache, visual changes, epigastric or right upper quadrant abdominal pain, nausea/vomiting, difficulty breathing, or decreased urine output. Although rapid weight gain and edema may raise the suspicion for preeclampsia, non-dependent edema is neither sensitive nor specific for preeclampsia and, therefore, no longer part of the diagnostic criteria. Laboratory testing is also useful in evaluating for end-organ involvement – including hemoglobin, platelet count, creatinine, and liver transaminases. Uric acid may also be helpful as it may identify a subgroup of hypertensive women at higher risk of premature delivery and small-for-gestational-age infants [27]. Fetal growth and well-being should be assessed using sonography to evaluate estimated fetal weight, progression of fetal growth, and amniotic fluid index. Non-stress testing and/or biophysical profiles may also be considered. Umbilical artery Doppler velocimetry may be helpful in the setting of FGR.

■ Management

Ongoing pregnancy management of GH should focus on close maternal and fetal monitoring for the development of preeclampsia, severe hypertension, maternal end-organ involvement, and/or fetal compromise. Management strategies to date are largely based on established practice patterns and expert opinion, rather than large clinical trials with clearly defined outcomes. One exception is the recently published HYPITAT trial [10] that addresses the issue of labor induction versus expectant management in the combined groups of gestational hypertensive or preeclamptic women.

Blood pressure is a key indicator in the disease process. As previously mentioned, blood pressure elevations should be sustained to establish the diagnosis of GH, and preeclampsia must be ruled out. The Pre-eclampsia Community Guideline (PRECOG) recommends that women with diastolic blood pressure between 90 and 99 mmHg, have blood tests to check for preeclampsia; if these are within normal ranges then blood pressure should be rechecked within seven days [2]. There have been no clinical trials to assess the effect of ambulatory blood pressure measurement vs. hospital measurement on maternal or fetal outcome [28]. However, ambulatory monitoring is an alternative strategy to repeated blood pressure measurement in the hospital setting and can serve to eliminate "white-coat" hypertension [29]. Using this ambulatory monitoring approach, only 38% of women were confirmed to actually have hypertension (defined as diastolic blood pressure > 85 mmHg in this study).

Women with mild GH should be given strict precautions to be watchful for and report any symptoms of preeclampsia, decreased fetal movement, and/or vaginal bleeding. In addition, weekly monitoring with blood pressure checks and urine protein evaluation are recommended. The frequency of subsequent laboratory testing may be tailored depending on the initial presentation, symptoms, severity of blood pressure, and any evidence of disease progression. Fetal surveillance with monitoring (one to two times per week non-stress tests and/or biophysical profile) should be considered. Growth ultrasounds should be performed once every three to four weeks with additional monitoring if there is any evidence of FGR.

Hospitalization

Hospitalization has been proposed for GH to reduce the progression to severe disease as well as to allow for rapid intervention in the event of abruption, eclampsia, or a hypertensive crisis. However, the evidence, including two randomized trials and a number of observational studies, suggest that women with mild GH can be managed safely at home or in a day-care facility [30–32]. Overall, perinatal complications are rare in women with mild GH and these women can be managed on an outpatient basis with well-defined precautions and surveillance. Furthermore, a randomized controlled trial of 54 women with GH demonstrated no difference in the use of antihypertensive drugs or pregnancy outcome between women who were managed as outpatients compared with inpatients. Inpatient management did not prevent the progression of GH to preeclampsia, but increased the likelihood of induction of labor [33]. This study suggests that inpatient management does not confer any benefit in the management of GH.

Bed rest

There is currently no evidence to support that complete or partial bed rest improves outcome in the setting of mild GH. Risks of bed rest during pregnancy including venous thromboembolism must also be considered.

Salt restriction

Based on a recent Cochrane review including two randomized trials, reduced salt intake does not appear to prevent progression to preeclampsia [34].

Medical therapy of hypertension

This is discussed in detail below. Medical therapy of mild hypertension has not been shown to improve neonatal outcomes [32] and may mask the diagnosis and recognition of progression to severe disease. Treatment should be considered with severe hypertension to prevent maternal cerebrovascular accidents.

Antenatal glucocorticoids

These are rarely indicated for mild GH as preterm delivery is not significantly higher than the general population. However, if there is evidence of progression to preeclampsia or severe GH suggesting the need for an indicated premature delivery, then glucocorticoids for fetal/neonatal benefit would be warranted.

Delivery timing

Severe GH at or near term is an indication for delivery. The timing of delivery for mild GH is less clear. As previously discussed, perinatal morbidity does not appear to be increased with mild GH. Some studies, however, possibly confounded by the heterogeneity of subjects included, suggest increased risk for pregnancy complications. Therefore, it is difficult to determine whether expectant management at term is a safe and reasonable option among women with GH. One study suggests that delivery between 39 and 40 weeks' gestation offers the lowest rate of adverse outcome in women with hypertensive disorders [35]. The HYPITAT trial addresses this issue of labor induction versus expectant management but combines GH with mild preeclampsia [10]. Maternal adverse outcomes including progression to severe hypertension are significantly reduced with induction of labor compared with expectant management without a difference in neonatal adverse outcomes after 37 weeks' gestation. There was no difference in Cesarean section rate between the induced and expectantly managed groups. Among women with GH alone, the relative risk of composite poor maternal outcomes was 0.81 (95% confidence interval, 0.63–1.03). Weighing the potential for progression to severe disease and associated risk for adverse maternal and neonatal outcomes against the favorable neonatal outcomes at term, our general approach is to deliver women with mild GH at term, but prior to 40 weeks' gestation.

■ Pharmacological treatment of GH

Pharmacological therapy of GH is reserved for severe hypertension, with the goal to reduce maternal complications such as cerebrovascular accidents. The CHIPS (Control of Hypertension in Pregnancy Study) pilot study indicated that a tight control of diastolic blood pressure (<85 mmHg) was associated with a lower incidence of severe hypertension and development of proteinuria. However, there was no statistically significant difference in severe complications or birthweight [36]. While the mean birthweight in the "tight control" group was 2501 g compared to 2675 g in the "less tight control" group, this study was not adequately powered in this regard. In another clinical trial from Egypt, 125 women with GH or preexisting hypertension were randomized to tight or less tight blood pressure control. Women in the tight blood pressure control group had a lower incidence of severe hypertension, and there was no difference in preterm birth or birthweight between the two groups [37]. Additional studies are planned to further explore whether tight blood pressure control in GH reduces maternal and perinatal morbidity.

There are several medications currently used for the treatment of GH. The agents used differ between the management of mild to moderate GH and severe GH. A Cochrane review of pharmacological agents used to treat severe GH found insufficient evidence to recommend one agent over another, and concluded that clinicians should use the agent with which they are most familiar [38], although in a small UK study 60–65% of practicing obstetricians and trainees were unable to name two side effects for their favored antihypertensive [39]. Therefore, clinicians must ensure that they are aware of the adverse effects of antihypertensive medications and the available alternatives. Currently, four main drugs are used in the management of GH: labetalol, methyldopa, nifedipine, and hydralazine. The latter is usually reserved for severe GH. A summary of the profile of these agents is shown in Table 6.1, the doses for acute and chronic management of GH are shown separately.

Labetalol

Labetalol is a mixed alpha- and beta-adrenergic antagonist. It is a well-tolerated antihypertensive that produces significant reduction in maternal blood pressure without any pronounced fetal effects [40]. Although

Drug	Use	Drug dose	Maximum dose	Important notes
Acute management of hypertension				
Labetalol	Antenatal, intrapartum, postpartum	200 mg orally If ineffective, loading dose 50 mg intravenously followed by infusion of 20–160 mg/h OR intermittent boluses 20–40 mg every 10–15 minutes intravenously	220 mg intravenously	Alpha- and beta-blocker, rapid onset of action Should be avoided in asthmatics
Nifedipine	Antenatal, intrapartum, postpartum	10 mg of oral form given (rapid onset) followed by 10–20 mg of modified-release form up to 8 hourly OR 10–20 mg orally every 30 minutes	50 mg orally	Rapid onset Sublingual form should not be given Side effects include headache
Hydralazine	Antenatal, intrapartum, postpartum	Loading dose 10–20 mg intravenously administered over 10–20 minutes, followed by intravenous infusion 1–5 mg/h OR intermittent intravenous boluses (5–10 mg every 20 minutes)	Maximum bolus dose 20 mg intravenously	Rapid onset of action Side effects of overdose similar to symptoms of severe preeclampsia, e.g., headache, tremors
Chronic management of hypertension				
Labetalol	Antenatal, intrapartum, postpartum	100 mg orally twice a day up to 600 mg four times a day	2400 mg/day	Alpha- and beta-blocker, rapid onset of action Should be avoided in asthmatics and patients with heart failure
Nifedipine	Antenatal, intrapartum, postpartum	10–20 mg orally up to three times a day OR long-acting form starting at 30 mg once a day	120 mg/day	Rapid onset Sublingual form should not be given Chronic side effects include headache and ankle edema
Methyldopa	Antenatal, postpartum	250 mg orally twice a day increasing up to 1 g four times a day	4 g/day	Slow onset of action, normally used to control preexisting hypertension or mild PIH Hemolysis may occur

Note: PIH, pregnancy-induced hypertension.

other beta-blockers have been tested, such as oxprenolol which has been compared with methyldopa, and atenolol compared with placebo; these have had varied success in the reduction of the risk of the development of preeclampsia [41,42]. Labetalol has replaced atenolol as the favored beta-blocker in pregnancy as it appears to have a less detrimental effect on fetal growth [43]. A small study has found no link between labetalol therapy and altered fetal behavior [44] and there is likewise no apparent association between labetalol administration and abnormalities of fetal heart rate [45]. For control of acute, severe GH, labetalol appears to be safer than hydralazine when both are administered intravenously [46]. However, due to its mode of action labetalol should not be used in patients with asthma or preexisting cardiac disease. Labetalol is safe during breast-feeding, but the infant should be monitored for evidence of bradycardia.

In pregnancy, dosing is typically initiated at 100 mg two to three times a day orally and can be increased to a maximum recommended dose of 2400 mg per day in split doses, e.g. 600 mg four times a day. For the control of severe GH, an intial dose of 200 mg can be given orally, if there is no response to this within 30 minutes, an intravenous dose of 50 mg over at least 1 minute can be given, followed by a maintenance infusion of 20 mg/h. Alternative dose regimens include intermittent boluses of intravenous labetalol, commencing with 10 mg, rising to 20–40 mg every 20 minutes until blood pressure is controlled. Labetalol can be diluted in 5% glucose or 0.9% sodium chloride for intravenous infusion.

Labetalol can induce hepatocellular damage which has been reported even with short-term use. This may be difficult to identify, as rising liver enzymes in maternal serum may also be a sign of worsening disease such as severe preeclampsia or HELLP (hemolysis, elevated liver enzymes, and low platelets) syndrome. An adverse reaction to labetalol should be considered when there is evidence of severe hepatocellular dysfunction in the absence of other signs of preeclampsia. Excessive doses of labetalol may also lead to maternal bradycardia. If this is severe leading to maternal hemodynamic compromise 600 μg of atropine sulfate can be given intravenously.

Nifedipine

Nifedipine is a calcium-channel antagonist, acting on L-type calcium channels which are present in the maternal vasculature and uterine smooth muscle (hence its alternative use as a tocolytic). Nifedipine is a potent antihypertensive, and should not be given sublingually as it can cause a precipitate fall in maternal blood pressure, which can lead to fetal distress [47] and has been associated with sudden death in an older cardiac population [48]. In contrast, oral long-acting nifedipine does not appear to have any adverse effects on the uteroplacental circulation or fetal heart rate [45]. Along with most other calcium-channel blockers nifedipine does not appear to be teratogenic [49] and is safe for breast-feeding women. Short-acting nifedipine reaches peak concentrations in maternal plasma after 40 minutes [50] and has an elimination half-life of approximately 80 minutes. Hence, short-acting nifedipine should be given every 4 hours to maintain therapeutic drug levels and efficacy [51]. Various modified-release formulations of nifedipine are available which have different clinical effects. There are currently no data to inform clinicians about the most effective way to deliver nifedipine when treating hypertension in pregnancy, as studies have used both short-acting and modified-release nifedipine [51,52]. In the UK, it is recommended that when prescribing modified-release nifedipine clinicians use the brand-name of the drug to prevent alterations in the medication dispensed and subsequent alterations in pharmacokinetics [53].

Due to its effects on cardiac afterload, nifedipine should be avoided in women with advanced aortic stenosis or impaired left ventricular function. The most commonly observed side effects are headache, edema, and palpitations. These may lead to concerns regarding progression to preeclampsia, which can be excluded by regular monitoring of urine for proteinuria. For the control of hypertension, nifedipine is usually commenced at 30 mg per day, which can be increased to 120 mg per day. Alternatively, 30 mg a day of extended-release nifedipine can be initiated with titration of the dose to achieve adequate blood pressure control. There is no evidence to determine whether administration once daily or split between two doses is preferable to control GH. However, it is hypothesized that a split dose regimen using a modified-release preparation would reduce fluctuation in maternal blood pressure.

Methyldopa

Methyldopa is a centrally acting antihypertensive, which is reflected in its side effect profile. Methyldopa remains a commonly used drug for long-term control of blood pressure in pregnancy. Methyldopa has been shown to improve fetal outcome when compared with placebo and is not associated with FGR [54]. Methyldopa does not appear to have any adverse effect on the uterine or feto-placental circulations [55,56] or the fetal heart rate [45]. There are long-term follow-up data at seven years which show no detriment to the offspring of women treated with methyldopa during pregnancy [57]. Methyldopa can have a depressant effect on the central nervous system, increasing tiredness and also reducing mental acuity. It should be used with caution in women with a history of depression. Methyldopa is excreted in breast milk, but the amount is too small to be harmful [53].

Methyldopa is given orally, commencing at 250 mg three times a day and increased gradually to a maximum dose of 1 g three times a day. Methyldopa is not suitable for rapid control of hypertension as it requires 24 hours to achieve therapeutic levels. As the dose of methyldopa increases the adverse effects, particularly sedation and depression, increase.

Hydralazine

Hydralazine, a direct-acting smooth muscle relaxant, is commonly used for acute blood pressure control with severe hypertension. The precise mode of action of hydralazine is unclear, but it is known to alter calcium balance in vascular cells [58] and promote hypoxia-inducible factors and vascular endothelial growth factor (VEGF) levels [59]. Intravenous boluses (5–20 mg over 10–20 minutes) will rapidly lower the blood pressure [60]. A recent meta-analysis, however, demonstrated that hydralazine was associated with significant increase in maternal hypotension, placental abruption, and a greater number of abnormal fetal heart rate recordings [46]. Therefore, it is probably best used as a second-line agent for women who do not have a sufficient antihypertensive response to labetalol.

During the intravenous bolus dose, blood pressure should be checked every 5 minutes. The drug may also then be given by continuous intravenous infusion between 1 and 5 mg/h. Side effects of hydralazine include headache, flushing, dizziness, and palpitations. These symptoms make differentiating between neurological progression of preeclampsia and common side effects of this medication problematic. Hydralazine is safe for breastfeeding mothers [53].

Pharmacological treatments not suitable for administration during pregnancy

Diuretics were formally used extensively for the "treatment" or prevention of preeclampsia. Meta-analysis has shown that while they reduce edema, these medications have no impact on perinatal survival [61]. Furosemide has significant effects throughout the cardiovascular system including: decreased cardiac output and stroke volume and increased peripheral resistance, but does not lower blood pressure [62]. Additionally, furosemide also reduces intervillous blood flow.

Angiotensin converting enzyme inhibitors and angiotensin receptor blockers are contraindicated in pregnancy as they are fetotoxic leading to fetal renal failure as evidenced by oligohydramnios antenatally and post-delivery as oliguria, and anuria [63]. Structural renal abnormalities and other dysmorphic features have also been reported [64].

Conclusion

Although GH shares many features with preeclampsia, there are important differences in the natural history of the disease processes. There are several important clinical questions that have yet to be answered, notably (1) whether treatment of mild GH prevents progression to severe GH or preeclampsia and (2) whether treatment poses any risk to the patient. The management of severe GH is similar to preeclampsia, with antihypertensive treatment indicated to reduce the risk of maternal cerebrovascular accidents. Close surveillance of women with GH is warranted to ensure that GH does not progress to preeclampsia or severe GH, which may have more serious consequences for both the mother and her fetus.

REFERENCES

1. Roberts JM, Pearson GD, Cutler JA, Lindheimer MD, National Heart Lung and Blood Institute. Summary of the NHLBI Working Group on Research on Hypertension During Pregnancy. *Hypertens Pregnancy.* 2003;**22**(2):109–27.

2. Milne F, Redman C, Walker J, *et al.* The pre-eclampsia community guideline (PRECOG): how to screen for and detect onset of pre-eclampsia in the community. *BMJ* 2005;**330**(7491):576–80.

3. Sibai BM, Caritis SN, Thom E, *et al.* Prevention of preeclampsia with low-dose aspirin in healthy, nulliparous pregnant women. The National Institute of Child Health and Human Development Network of Maternal-Fetal Medicine Units. *N Engl J Med* 1993;**329**(17):1213–18.

4. Knuist M, Bonsel GJ, Zondervan HA, Treffers PE. Intensification of fetal and maternal surveillance in pregnant women with hypertensive disorders. *Int J Gynaecol Obstet* 1998;**61**(2):127–33.

5. Hauth JC, Ewell MG, Levine RJ, *et al.* Pregnancy outcomes in healthy nulliparas who developed hypertension. Calcium for Preeclampsia Prevention Study Group. *Obstet Gynecol* 2000;**95**(1):24–8.

6. Campbell DM, MacGillivray I. Preeclampsia in twin pregnancies: incidence and outcome. *Hypertens Pregnancy* 1999;**18**(3):197–207.

7. Sibai BM, Hauth J, Caritis S, *et al.* Hypertensive disorders in twin versus singleton gestations. *Am J Obstet Gynecol* 2000;**182**(4):938–42.

8. Barton JR, O'Brien JM, Bergauer NK, Jacques DL, Sibai BM. Mild gestational hypertension remote from term: progression and outcome. *Am J Obstet Gynecol* 2001;**184**(5):979–83.

9. Saudan P, Brown MA, Buddle ML, Jones M. Does gestational hypertension become pre-eclampsia? *Br J Obstet Gynaecol* 1998;**105**(11):1177–84.

10. Koopmans CM, Bijlenga D, Groen H, *et al.* Induction of labor versus expectant monitoring for gestational hypertension or mild pre-eclampsia after 36 weeks' gestation (HYPITAT): a multicentre, open-label randomised controlled trial. *Lancet* 2009;**374**(9694):979–88.

11. Sibai BM. Diagnosis and management of gestational hypertension and preeclampsia. *Obstet Gynecol* 2003;**102**(1):181–92.

12. Buchbinder A, Sibai BM, Caritis S, *et al.* Adverse perinatal outcomes are significantly higher in severe gestational hypertension than in mild preeclampsia. *Am J Obstet Gynecol* 2002;**186**(1):66–71.

13. Knutzen VK, Davey DA. Hypertension in pregnancy and perinatal mortality. *S Afr Med J* 1977;**51**(19):675–9.

14. Stella CL, O'Brien JM, Forrester KJ, *et al.* The coexistence of gestational hypertension and diabetes: influence on pregnancy outcome. *Am J Perinatol* 2008;**25**(6):325–9.

15. Pijnenborg R, Anthony J, Davey DA, *et al.* Placental bed spiral arteries in the hypertensive disorders of pregnancy. *Br J Obstet Gynaecol* 1991;**98**(7):648–55.

16. Becroft DM, Thompson JM, Mitchell EA. Placental infarcts, intervillous fibrin plaques, and intervillous thrombi: incidences, cooccurrences, and epidemiological associations. *Pediatr Dev Pathol* 2004;**7**(1):26–34.

17. Koenig JM, Chegini N. Enhanced expression of Fas-associated proteins in decidual and trophoblastic tissues in pregnancy-induced hypertension. *Am J Reprod Immunol* 2000;**44**(6):347–9.

18. Nicolaides KH, Faratian B, Symonds EM. Effect on low implantation of the placenta on maternal blood pressure and placental function. *Br J Obstet Gynaecol* 1982;**89**(10):806–10.

19. Ananth CV, Bowes WA, Jr., Savitz DA, Luther ER. Relationship between pregnancy-induced hypertension and placenta previa: a population-based study. *Am J Obstet Gynecol* 1997;**177**(5):997–1002.

20. Nemeth I, Talosi G, Papp A, Boda D. Xanthine oxidase activation in mild gestational hypertension. *Hypertens Pregnancy* 2002;**21**(1):1–11.

21. Strevens H, Wide-Swensson D, Hansen A, *et al.* Glomerular endotheliosis in normal pregnancy and pre-eclampsia. *BJOG* 2003;**110**(9):831–6.

22. Villar J, Carroli G, Wojdyla D, *et al.* Preeclampsia, gestational hypertension and intrauterine growth restriction, related or independent conditions? *Am J Obstet Gynecol* 2006;**194**(4):921–31.

23. Zafirovska KG, Maleska VT, Bogdanovska SV, *et al.* Plasma human atrial natriuretic peptide, endothelin-1, aldosterone and plasma-renin activity in pregnancy-induced hypertension. *J Hypertens* 1999;**17**(9):1317–22.

24. Lee MI, Bottoms SF, Sokol RJ, Todd HM. Angiotensin converting enzyme activity in hypertensive pregnancy. *J Perinat Med* 1987;**15**(3):258–62.

25. Nalogowska-Glosnicka K, Lacka BI, Zychma MJ, *et al.* Angiotensin II type 1 receptor gene A1166C polymorphism is associated with the increased risk of pregnancy-induced hypertension. *Med Sci Monit* 2000;**6**(3):523–9.

26. Meagher EA, FitzGerald GA. Disordered eicosanoid formation in pregnancy-induced hypertension. *Circulation* 1993;**88**(3):1324–33.

27. Roberts JM, Bodnar LM, Lain KY, *et al.* Uric acid is as important as proteinuria in identifying fetal risk in women with gestational hypertension.[see comment]. *Hypertension* 2005;**46**(6):1263–9.

28. Bergel E, Carroli G, Althabe F. Ambulatory versus conventional methods for monitoring blood pressure during pregnancy. *Cochrane Database Syst Rev* 2002;(2):CD001231.

29. Biswas A, Choolani MA, Anandakumar C, Arulkumaran S. Ambulatory blood pressure monitoring in pregnancy induced hypertension. *Acta Obstet Gynecol Scand* 1997;**76**(9):829–33.

30. Mathews DD, Agarwal V, Shuttleworth TP. The effect of rest and ambulation on plasma urea and urate levels in pregnant women with proteinuric hypertension. *Br J Obstet Gynaecol* 1980;**87**(12):1095–8.

31. Crowther CA, Bouwmeester AM, Ashurst HM. Does admission to hospital for bed rest prevent disease progression or improve fetal outcome in pregnancy complicated by non-proteinuric hypertension? *Br J Obstet Gynaecol* 1992;**99**(1):13–17.

32. Barton JR, Witlin AG, Sibai BM. Management of mild preeclampsia. *Clin Obstet Gynecol* 1999;**42**(3):455–69.

33. Tuffnell DJ, Lilford RJ, Buchan PC, *et al.* Randomised controlled trial of day care for hypertension in pregnancy. *Lancet* 1992;**339**(8787):224–7.

34. Duley L, Henderson-Smart D, Meher S. Altered dietary salt for preventing pre-eclampsia, and its complications. *Cochrane Database Syst Rev* 2005;(4):CD005548.

35. Nicholson JM, Kellar LC, Kellar GM. The impact of the interaction between increasing gestational age and obstetrical risk on birth outcomes: evidence of a varying optimal time of delivery. *J Perinatol* 2006;**26**(7):392–402.

36. Magee LA, von Dadelszen P, Chan S, *et al.* The Control of Hypertension In Pregnancy Study pilot trial. *BJOG* 2007;**114**(6):770, e13–20.

37. El Guindy AA, Nabhan AF. A randomized trial of tight vs. less tight control of mild essential and gestational hypertension in pregnancy. *J Perinat Med* 2008;**36**(5):413–18.

38. Duley L, Henderson-Smart DJ. Drugs for treatment of very high blood pressure during pregnancy. *Cochrane Database Syst Rev* 2002;(4):CD001449.

39. Heazell AEP, Mahomoud S, Pirie AM. Current knowledge and practice in treatment of severe acute hypertension in pregnancy – an audit of practice in West Midlands obstetric units. *J Obstet Gynaecol* 2004;**24**(8):897–8.

40. Pickles CJ, Symonds EM, Broughton Pipkin F. The fetal outcome in a randomized double-blind controlled trial of labetalol versus placebo in pregnancy-induced hypertension. *Br J Obstet Gynaecol* 1989;**96**(1):38–43.

41. Gallery ED, Saunders DM, Hunyor SN, Gyory AZ. Randomised comparison of methyldopa and oxprenolol for treatment of hypertension in pregnancy. *Br Med J* 1979;**1**(6178):1591–4.

42. Rubin PC, Low RA, Reid JL. Antihypertensive therapy in pregnancy. *Lancet* 1983;**1**(8334):1160.

43. Butters L, Kennedy S, Rubin PC. Atenolol in essential hypertension during pregnancy. *BMJ* 1990;**301**(6752):587–9.

44. Gazzolo D, Visser GH, Santi F, *et al.* Behavioural development and Doppler velocimetry in relation to perinatal outcome in small for dates fetuses. *Early Hum Dev* 1995;**43**(2):185–95.

45. Waterman EJ, Magee LA, Lim KI, *et al.* Do commonly used oral antihypertensives alter fetal or neonatal heart rate characteristics? A systematic review. *Hypertens Pregnancy* 2004;**23**(2):155–69.

46. Magee LA, Cham C, Waterman EJ, Ohlsson A, von Dadelszen P. Hydralazine for treatment of severe hypertension in pregnancy: meta-analysis. *BMJ* 2003; **327**(7421):955–60.

47. Impey L. Severe hypotension and fetal distress following sublingual administration of nifedipine to a patient with severe pregnancy induced hypertension at 33 weeks. *Br J Obstet Gynaecol* 1993;**100**:959–61.

48. Grossman E, Messerli FH, Grodzicki T, Kowey P. Should a moratorium be placed on sublingual nifedipine capsules given for hypertensive emergencies and pseudoemergencies?[see comment]. *JAMA* 1996;**276**(16):1328–31.

49. Magee LA, Schick B, Donnenfeld AE, *et al.* The safety of calcium channel blockers in human pregnancy: a prospective, multicenter cohort study. *Am J Obstet Gynecol* 1996;**174**(3):823–8.

50. Prevost RR, Akl SA, Whybrew WD, Sibai BM. Oral nifedipine pharmacokinetics in pregnancy-induced hypertension. *Pharmacotherapy* 1992;**12**(3):174–7.

51. Barton JR, Prevost RR, Wilson DA, Whybrew WD, Sibai BM. Nifedipine pharmacokinetics and pharmacodynamics during the immediate postpartum period in patients with preeclampsia. *Am J Obstet Gynecol* 1991;**165**(4 Pt 1): 951–4.

52. Gruppo di Studio Ipertensione in Gravidanza. Nifedipine versus expectant management in mild to moderate hypertension in pregnancy. *Br J Obstet Gynaecol* 1998;**105**(7):718–22.

53. Royal Pharmaceutical Society of Great Britain. *British National Fomulary.* London, BMJ and Royal Pharmaceutical Society, 2009.

54. Redman CW. Fetal outcome in trial of antihypertensive treatment in pregnancy. *Lancet* 1976;**2**(7989):753–6.

55. Montan S, Anandakumar C, Arulkumaran S, Ingemarsson I, Ratnam SS. Effects of methyldopa on uteroplacental and fetal hemodynamics in pregnancy-induced hypertension. *Am J Obstet Gynecol* 1993;**168**(1 Pt 1):152–6.

56. Houlihan DD, Dennedy MC, Ravikumar N, Morrison JJ. Anti-hypertensive therapy and the feto-placental circulation: effects on umbilical artery resistance. *J Perinat Med* 2004;**32**(4):315–19.

57. Cockburn J, Moar VA, Ounsted M, Redman CW. Final report of study on hypertension during pregnancy: the effects of specific treatment on the growth and development of the children. *Lancet* 1982;**1**(8273):647–9.

58. Jacobs M. Mechanism of action of hydralazine on vascular smooth muscle. *Biochem Pharmacol* 1984;**33**(18):2915–19.

59. Knowles HJ, Tian YM, Mole DR, Harris AL. Novel mechanism of action for hydralazine: induction of hypoxia-inducible factor-1alpha, vascular endothelial growth factor, and angiogenesis by inhibition of prolyl hydroxylases. *Circ Res* 2004;**95**(2):162–9.

60. Paterson-Brown S, Robson SC, Redfern N, Walkinshaw SA, de Swiet M. Hydralazine boluses for the treatment of severe hypertension in pre-eclampsia. *Br J Obstet Gynaecol* 1994;**101**(5):409–13.

61. Collins R, Chalmers I, Peto R. Antihypertensive treatment in pregnancy. *Br Med J (Clin Res Ed)* 1985;**291**(6502):1129.

62. Carr DB, Gavrila D, Brateng D, Easterling TR. Maternal hemodynamic changes associated with furosemide treatment. *Hypertens Pregnancy* 2007;**26**(2):173–8.

63. Laube GF, Kemper MJ, Schubiger G, Neuhaus TJ. Angiotensin-converting enzyme inhibitor fetopathy: long-term outcome. *Arch Dis Child Fetal Neonatal Ed* 2007;**92**(5):F402–3.

64. Serreau R, Luton D, Macher MA, *et al.* Developmental toxicity of the angiotensin II type 1 receptor antagonists during human pregnancy: a report of 10 cases. *BJOG* 2005;**112**(6):710–12.

Secondary hypertension in pregnancy

Fergus P. McCarthy and Louise C. Kenny

7

■ Introduction

Most forms of hypertension have no known underlying cause and are known as "essential hypertension" or "primary hypertension." However, in approximately 10% of the cases, there is a known cause, and thus the hypertension is referred to as secondary hypertension. Blood pressure falls in the first and second trimesters of pregnancy. Therefore, women with high blood pressure before the 20th week of pregnancy are assumed to have preexisting hypertension which may be essential or secondary hypertension. As many women of reproductive age only present for the first time when pregnant, chronic hypertension is often revealed in the first half of pregnancy. In women presenting with hypertension in the first half of pregnancy it is important to look for an underlying cause. Many of these disorders can be cured, leading to partial or complete normalization of the blood pressure. However, it is not cost-effective to perform a complete evaluation of every hypertensive patient, therefore it is important to assess the patient for signs and symptoms that suggest the possibility of secondary hypertension.

There are many causes of secondary hypertension and these are summarized in Table 7.1. Many of the disorders listed in this table are common (e.g., renal disease) while others are extremely rare (e.g., pheochromocytoma). Nevertheless, it is important for the obstetrician to be aware of them all and to able to undertake basic steps to exclude them, either on clinical grounds or by more detailed investigation (Table 7.2). Consideration is given here to the more significant causes of secondary hypertension in the pregnant patient.

Hypertension in Pregnancy, ed. Alexander Heazell, Errol R. Norwitz, Louise C. Kenny, and Philip N. Baker. Published by Cambridge University Press. © Cambridge University Press 2010.

Table 7.1 Secondary causes of hypertension

Group	Condition
Renovascular hypertension	
Hypertension secondary to other renal disorders	Polycystic kidney disease
	Nephritic and nephrotic syndrome
	Chronic glomerulonephritis
	Reflux nephropathy
	Diabetic nephropathy
Hypertension secondary to connective tissue disorders	Rheumatoid disease
	Systemic lupus erythematosus
	Polyarteritis nodosa
	Systemic sclerosis
	Scleroderma
Hypertension secondary to endocrine disorders	Pheochromocytoma
	Hyperaldosteronism
	Cushing's syndrome
	Hyperparathyroidism
	Acromegaly
	Hyperthyroidism
	Hypothyroidism
Hypertension secondary to cardiovascular disorders	Malformed aorta
	Aortic valve disease
	Neurofibromatosis
	Coarctation of the aorta
Drugs causing secondary hypertension	Steroid use
	Heavy alcohol consumption
	In particular, alcohol, nasal decongestants with adrenergic effects, non-steroidal anti-inflammatory drugs, monoamine oxidase inhibitors, adrenoceptor stimulants, and combined methods of hormonal contraception (those containing ethinyl-estradiol)
Other causes of secondary hypertension	Obstructive sleep apnoea
	Fever
	Neoplasms
	Anemia

■ Renal system causes of secondary hypertension

Renovascular disease

Renovascular disease is a general term used for three disorders which result in renovascular occlusion; renal artery stenosis, renal vein

Table 7.2 Clinical findings in causes of secondary hypertension

System affected	Disorder	Possible clinical findings/clues
Vascular system	Renovascular hypertension	Sudden onset <30 years of age
		No family history or other risk factors for hypertension
		Resistant to antihypertensives
		A systolic–diastolic abdominal bruit
	Aortic coarctation	Hypertension in the upper extremities
		Reduced or delayed femoral pulses
		Low or unobtainable arterial blood pressure in the lower extremities
Endocrine system	Diabetes mellitus	Fasting plasma glucose ≥ 140 mg/dL (7.8 mmol/L) or a two-hour glucose ≥ 200 mg/dL (11.1 mmol/L) [1]
	Hyperthyroidism	Low serum thyroid-stimulating hormone, High free thyroxine (T4) and triiodothyronine (T3)
	Hypothyroidism	High serum thyroid-stimulating hormone
	Hyperparathyroidism	Unexplained hypercalcemia causing "stones, bones, abdominal groans" i.e., anorexia, nausea, vomiting, bone pain, osteoporosis, kidney stones, confusion, and fatigue
	Pheochromocytoma	Paroxysmal elevations in blood pressure Associated with headache, palpitations, and sweating
	Acromegaly	Elevated insulin-like growth factor 1 (IGF-1) followed by oral glucose tolerance test with growth hormone levels
	Cushing's syndrome	Cushingoid facies, central obesity, proximal muscle weakness, and ecchymoses
	Primary hyperaldosteronism	Unexplained hypokalemia

thrombosis, and renal atheroembolism. However, the term generally refers to renal artery disease as the other two disorders are uncommon. In renal artery stenosis, occlusion of the renal artery results in renal ischemia which causes hypertension due to activation of the renin–angiotensin system. Renovascular disease is generally a disorder of older men secondary to atherosclerosis. However, a specific type of renovascular occlusion may occur in younger women and this is called fibromuscular dysplasia (FMD). Fibromuscular dysplasia is a non-inflammatory, non-atherosclerotic disorder that leads to arterial stenosis and typically involves the distal two thirds and branches of the renal arteries. It occurs bilaterally in the renal arteries in 30–50% of cases but may occur in other arterial beds [2,3].

Several factors are associated with a higher likelihood of hypertension occurring secondary to renovascular disease. These include the onset of hypertension under the age of 30 occurring in the absence of any family history of hypertension and other risk factors for hypertension such as diabetes and obesity, hypertension resistant to multiple therapeutic doses of antihypertensive agents, and an acute rise in blood pressure over a previously stable baseline in patients with previously well-controlled hypertension [4].

The gold standard for diagnosis of renovascular disease is renal arteriography but this is contraindicated in pregnancy. Magnetic resonance angiography is increasingly used as a first-line screening test for renovascular hypertension [5]. Duplex Doppler ultrasonography is an alternative diagnostic modality but is technically difficult and time-consuming [6]. It is important to recognize renovascular disease as a cause of secondary hypertension as it is potentially correctable. Percutaneous transluminal angioplasty has generally replaced surgery in the management of renal artery stenosis [7]. However, some patients will be managed pharmacologically using medications such as angiotensin converting enzyme (ACE) inhibitors, but ACE inhibitors are contraindicated in pregnancy.

Primary renal disease

Women with underlying renal disease are at significantly increased risk of poor pregnancy outcome and require multidisciplinary care. In pregnant women with underlying renal disease, proteinuria worsens in approximately half and hypertension worsens in approximately a quarter of cases [8,9]. In patients with preexisting renal disease, the risk of renal function deterioration throughout the course of pregnancy varies depending on the initial pre-pregnancy level of impairment.

In women with mild renal impairment (plasma creatinine concentration less than 1.5mg/dL or 132μmol/L), pregnancy is associated with a permanent decline in renal function in between 0% and 10% of women.

In women with moderate renal impairment (plasma creatinine concentration between 1.5 and 2.9mg/dL or 132 and 255μmol/L) the plasma creatinine concentration tends to decline modestly during the first half of pregnancy and then may rise above the previous baseline as the pregnancy progresses. In women with severe renal impairment (plasma creatinine concentration above 3mg/dL or 265μmol/L) conception is unlikely due to amenorrhea or anovulation. The underlying cause of the renal disease does not appear to be the major determinant of worsening renal disease (excluding lupus nephritis). An elevated plasma creatinine concentration (above 1.5mg/dL or 132μmol/L) and hypertension are the major risk factors for permanent exacerbation of underlying renal disease.

A detailed review of all causes of primary renal disease and their effects on pregnancy is outside the scope of this chapter. Generally, women with renal disease in pregnancy should have the following:

- Increased frequency of antenatal visits occurring every two weeks until the third trimester and then weekly until delivery;
- Early detection and treatment of asymptomatic bacteriuria;
- At least monthly monitoring of maternal renal function (plasma urea, creatinine, and electrolytes, urinary protein:creatinine ratios);
- Monitoring for the development of preeclampsia;
- Timely treatment of maternal hypertension;
- Fetal surveillance with ultrasound to assess fetal growth at least every four weeks. If fetal growth restriction (FGR) is detected, ultrasound surveillance should increase to fortnightly growth assessments with weekly umbilical artery Doppler and amniotic fluid index measurements.
- Multidisciplinary care to ensure a timely delivery while minimizing fetal prematurity. Preterm intervention may be necessary in the presence of deteriorating renal function, severe preeclampsia, FGR or a non-reassuring fetal state.

■ Vascular system causes of secondary hypertension

Coarctation of the aorta

Coarctation of the aorta is a form of a congenital heart defect and may occur in isolation or in conjunction with other cardiac defects such as a bicuspid aortic valve or ventricular septal defect [10]. Coarctation of the aorta comprises 5–8% of all congenital heart defects and may be defined as a constricted aortic segment that comprises localized medial thickening, with some infolding of the medial and superimposed neointimal tissue. It is thought to occur either as the result of a developmental problem due to reduced intrauterine blood flow causing underdevelopment of the aortic arch or due to the constriction of ductal tissue extending into the thoracic aorta [11–13]. The coarctation may be discrete, or a long segment of the aorta may be narrowed. The former is more common. The classical coarctation is located in the thoracic aorta distal to the origin of the left subclavian artery at approximately the level of the ductal structure. The condition is usually diagnosed in early childhood when children present with symptoms of congestive heart failure but coarctation may also present with hypertension in older children and adults. Patients presenting later in life often do not have congestive heart failure due to the presence of arterial collateral vessels. The classical clinical findings in patients with coarctation of the aorta are hypertension in the upper extremities, delayed or reduced brachiofemoral pulses, and low or unobtainable blood pressure in the lower extremities. The diagnosis can be confirmed using echocardiography or magnetic resonance imaging techniques. Women with a repaired and unrepaired coarctation appear to have a higher incidence of miscarriage and preeclampsia in pregnancy [14,15]. Major complications associated with unrepaired coarctation of the aorta in pregnancy are uncommon but include dissection of the aorta, intracranial hemorrhage, and left ventricular heart failure [16].

■ Endocrine system causes of secondary hypertension

Pheochromocytoma

Pheochromocytomas are catecholamine-producing tumor that arise from chromaffin cells of the adrenal medulla or the sympathetic ganglia (also known as extra-adrenal pheochromocytomas). Pheochromocytomas are rare with an annual incidence of two to eight cases per one million people and an estimated prevalence in unselected patients with hypertension of 0.2% to 0.6%.

Pregnancy is extremely hazardous in women with pheochromocytoma. It often mimics preeclampsia in its presentation and is therefore frequently diagnosed late. Undiagnosed and inappropriately treated pheochromocytomas are associated with high rates of both fetal and maternal mortality. However, the majority of evidence regarding pheochromocytoma and pregnancy originates from case reports and case series [17]. The classic triad of symptoms in patients with a pheochromocytoma consists of episodic headache, sweating, and tachycardia [18]. Approximately half the patients with pheochromocytoma have paroxysmal hypertension. The other half have what appears to be essential hypertension.

The diagnostic approach to catecholamine-producing tumor is divided into two stages. First, the diagnosis of a catecholamine-producing tumor must be suspected and then confirmed biochemically by increased concentrations of fractionated metanephrines and catecholamines in the urine. The next step is to localize the catecholamine-producing tumor to guide the surgical approach. About 98% of catecholamine-producing tumor are located in the abdomen and pelvis, with approximately 90% of them in the adrenal glands. Magnetic resonance imaging is the localization test of choice in pregnancy. Stimulation tests, such as the clonidine suppression test, and other tests such as [123]-I-metaiodobenzylguanidine scintigraphy are not considered safe for pregnant women. Although some controversy exists about the most appropriate management, pheochromocytomas should be removed promptly if diagnosed during the first two trimesters of pregnancy. If the patient is in the third trimester, Cesarean section and removal of the pheochromocytoma in the same operation are indicated [19]. Spontaneous labor and delivery should be avoided [20].

Primary hyperaldosteronism

Primary hyperaldosteronism is characterized by hypertension, hypokalaemia, suppressed plasma renin activity, and increased aldosterone excretion. Bilateral idiopathic hyperaldosteronism (IHA) and aldosterone-producing adenoma (APA) are the most common subtypes of primary hyperaldosteronism. A much less common form, unilateral hyperplasia or primary adrenal hyperplasia, is caused by zona glomerulosa hyperplasia of predominantly one adrenal gland [21]. Two forms of familial hyperaldosteronism (FH) have been described: FH type I and FH type II. Familial hyperaldosteronism type I, or glucocorticoid-remediable hyperaldosteronism, is a rare autosomal dominant form and is suppressible with exogenous glucocorticoids, and FH type II refers to the familial occurrence of APA or IHA or both.

Primary hyperaldosteronism is a relatively common form of secondary hypertension, affecting 5–10% of all patients with hypertension. Plasma and urinary aldosterone levels increase markedly in pregnancy so absolute levels are of limited value in establishing the diagnosis. The diagnosis of primary hyperaldosteronism may be confirmed by aldosterone suppression testing with sodium loading and volume expansion (oral sodium loading, saline suppression test, or fludrocortisone suppression testing). The goals of therapy for primary hyperaldosteronism due to either unilateral or bilateral adrenal disease are the same and include normalization of the serum potassium in hypokalemic patients, normalization of the blood pressure, and reversal of the adverse cardiovascular effects of hyperaldosteronism [22]. Provided that blood pressure is controlled and that the serum potassium is normalized, pregnancy appears to be relatively uncomplicated and definitive subtype evaluation and treatment can be delayed until the postpartum period.

Cushing's syndrome

Cushing's syndrome during pregnancy is a rare condition with fewer than 150 cases reported in the literature [23]. Cushing's syndrome in pregnancy is rare due to the fact that untreated Cushing's syndrome is associated with a high prevalence ($>75\%$) of ovulatory dysfunction secondary to cortisol excess [24]. The etiology of Cushing's syndrome differs between the pregnant and non-pregnant state. Adrenal adenomas underlie a disproportionately high proportion of cases in pregnancy accounting for approximately 40–50% of cases in comparison with 17–29% in non-pregnant women. Conversely, Cushing's disease appears to be less common in pregnancy, with rates of 63–72% in the general population, compared with approximately 33% in pregnant women.

Pregnancy dramatically affects the maternal hypothalamic–pituitary–adrenal axis, resulting in increased hepatic production of corticosteroid-binding globulin, increased levels of serum, salivary, and urinary free cortisol, lack of suppression of cortisol levels after dexamethasone administration, and placental production of corticotropin releasing hormone (CRH) and adrenocorticotropic hormone (ACTH). Moreover, a blunted response of ACTH and cortisol to exogenous CRH may also occur. Therefore, the diagnosis of Cushing's syndrome during pregnancy is much more difficult.

Misdiagnosis is also common, as the syndrome may be easily confused with preeclampsia or gestational diabetes. Signs and symptoms that occur in Cushing's syndrome such as weight gain, striae, and hypertension are also common in pregnancy. Because Cushing's syndrome during pregnancy is usually associated with severe maternal and fetal complications, its early diagnosis and treatment are critical. In pregnancy the fetus is partially protected from the hypercortisolemia because 85% of maternal cortisol is converted to biologically inactive cortisone by placental 11-beta-hydroxysteroid dehydrogenase. Untreated Cushing's syndrome has been associated with spontaneous miscarriage, premature delivery, and, rarely, neonatal adrenal insufficiency. Surgery is the treatment of choice for Cushing's syndrome in pregnancy, except perhaps in the late third trimester, with medical therapy being a second choice. There does not seem to be a rationale for supportive treatment alone.

■ Other causes of secondary hypertension

Medications, drugs, and alcohol

Oral contraceptives, non-steroidal anti-inflammatory drugs, alcohol abuse, and a variety of antidepressants, such as those acting on noradrenergic and serotonergic systems, have been associated with the development of secondary hypertension [25].

REFERENCES

1. Alberti KG, Zimmet PZ. Definition, diagnosis and classification of diabetes mellitus and its complications. Part 1: diagnosis and classification of diabetes mellitus provisional report of a WHO consultation. *Diabet Med* 1998;**15**(7):539–53.
2. Estepa R, Gallego N, Orte L, *et al.* Renovascular hypertension in children. *Scand J Urol Nephrol* 2001;**35**(5):388–92.
3. Luscher TF, Keller HM, Imhof HG, *et al.* Fibromuscular hyperplasia: extension of the disease and therapeutic outcome. Results of the University Hospital Zurich Cooperative Study on Fibromuscular Hyperplasia. *Nephron* 1986;**44** Suppl 1:109–14.

4. Hirsch AT, Haskal ZJ, Hertzer NR, *et al.* ACC/AHA 2005 Practice Guidelines for the management of patients with peripheral arterial disease (lower extremity, renal, mesenteric, and abdominal aortic): a collaborative report from the American Association for Vascular Surgery/Society for Vascular Surgery, Society for Cardiovascular Angiography and Interventions, Society for Vascular Medicine and Biology, Society of Interventional Radiology, and the ACC/AHA Task Force on Practice Guidelines (Writing Committee to Develop Guidelines for the Management of Patients With Peripheral Arterial Disease): endorsed by the American Association of Cardiovascular and Pulmonary Rehabilitation; National Heart, Lung, and Blood Institute; Society for Vascular Nursing; TransAtlantic Inter-Society Consensus; and Vascular Disease Foundation. *Circulation* 2006;**113**(11):e463–654.

5. Postma CT, Joosten FB, Rosenbusch G, Thien T. Magnetic resonance angiography has a high reliability in the detection of renal artery stenosis. *Am J Hypertens* 1997;**10**(9 Pt 1):957–63.

6. Leung DA, Hoffmann U, Pfammatter T, *et al.* Magnetic resonance angiography versus duplex sonography for diagnosing renovascular disease. *Hypertension* 1999;**33**(2):726–31.

7. Tullis MJ, Caps MT, Zierler RE, *et al.* Blood pressure, antihypertensive medication, and atherosclerotic renal artery stenosis. *Am J Kidney Dis* 1999;**33**(4):675–81.

8. Bar J, Ben-Rafael Z, Padoa A, *et al.* Prediction of pregnancy outcome in subgroups of women with renal disease. *Clin Nephrol* 2000;**53**(6):437–44.

9. Hou S, Pregnancy in chronic renal insufficiency and end-stage renal disease. *Am J Kidney Dis* 1999;**33**(2):235–52.

10. Nihoyannopoulos P, Karas S, Sapsford RN, Hallidie-Smith K, Foale R. Accuracy of two-dimensional echocardiography in the diagnosis of aortic arch obstruction. *J Am Coll Cardiol* 1987;**10**(5):1072–7.

11. Rudolph AM, Heymann MA, Spitznas U. Hemodynamic considerations in the development of narrowing of the aorta. *Am J Cardiol* 1972;**30**(5):514–25.

12. Talner NS, Berman MA. Postnatal development of obstruction in coarctation of the aorta: role of the ductus arteriosus. *Pediatrics* 1975;**56**(4):562–9.

13. Wielenga G, Dankmeijer J. Coarctation of the aorta. *J Pathol Bacteriol* 1968;**95**(1):265–74.

14. Vriend JW, Drenthen W, Pieper PG, *et al.* Outcome of pregnancy in patients after repair of aortic coarctation. *Eur Heart J* 2005;**26**(20):2173–8.

15. Drenthen W, Pieper PG, Roos-Hesselink JW, *et al.* Outcome of pregnancy in women with congenital heart disease: a literature review. *J Am Coll Cardiol* 2007;**49**(24):2303–11.

16. Beauchesne LM, Connolly HM, Ammash NM, Warnes CA. Coarctation of the aorta: outcome of pregnancy. *J Am Coll Cardiol* 2001;**38**(6):1728–33.

17. Almog B, Kuperminc MJ, Many A, Lessing JB. Pheochromocytoma in pregnancy–a case report and review of the literature. *Acta Obstet Gynecol Scand* 2000; **79**(8):709–11.

18. Stein PP, Black HR. A simplified diagnostic approach to pheochromocytoma. A review of the literature and report of one institution's experience. *Medicine (Baltimore)* 1991;**70**(1):46–66.

19. Takahashi K, Sai Y, Nosaka S. Anaesthetic management for caesarean section combined with removal of pheochromocytoma. *Eur J Anaesthesiol* 1998;**15**(3): 364–6.

20. Stenstrom G, Swolin K. Pheochromocytoma in pregnancy. Experience of treatment with phenoxybenzamine in three patients. *Acta Obstet Gynecol Scand* 1985;**64**(4):357–61.

21. Mattsson C, Young WF, Jr. Primary aldosteronism: diagnostic and treatment strategies. *Nat Clin Pract Nephrol* 2006;**2**(4):198–208; quiz, 1 p following 230.

22. Funder JW, Carey RM, Fardella C, *et al.* Case detection, diagnosis, and treatment of patients with primary aldosteronism: an endocrine society clinical practice guideline. *J Clin Endocrinol Metab* 2008;**93**(9):3266–81.

23. Lindsay JR, Jonklaas J, Oldfield EH, Nieman LK. Cushing's syndrome during pregnancy: personal experience and review of the literature. *J Clin Endocrinol Metab* 2005;**90**(5):3077–83.

24. Buescher MA, McClamrock HD, Adashi EY. Cushing syndrome in pregnancy. *Obstet Gynecol* 1992;**79**(1):130–7.

25. Licht CM, de Geus EJ, Seldenrijk A, *et al.* Depression is associated with decreased blood pressure, but antidepressant use increases the risk for hypertension. *Hypertension* 2009;**53**(4):631–8.

Identification, diagnosis, and management of suspected preeclampsia

8

Fiona Milne and Philip N. Baker on behalf of the PRECOG (Pre-eclampsia Community Guideline) development group

■ Introduction

Preeclampsia is responsible for a third of severe obstetric morbidity and remains a leading cause of maternal and fetal death [1]. Issues of substandard care in the management of preeclampsia include failures to identify and act on known risk factors at booking and to recognize and respond to signs and symptoms of preeclampsia from 20 weeks' gestation [2]. The PRECOG group, under the auspices of Action on Pre-eclampsia, have developed these recommendations for the screening and detection of preeclampsia [3,4] (www.apec.org.uk/guidelines.htm). They provide an evidence-based risk assessment, a list of factors suitable for the identification of, early referral, a two-tier schedule of assessment and a step-up referral, and assessment for signs of preeclampsia. These recommendations and the supporting evidence, which we discuss in this chapter, are relevant to antenatal care worldwide, as local circumstances and needs dictate.

Hypertension in Pregnancy, ed. Alexander Heazell, Errol R. Norwitz, Louise C. Kenny, and Philip N. Baker. Published by Cambridge University Press. © Cambridge University Press 2010.

■ Definitions used in this chapter

Hypertension – A diastolic blood pressure of 90 mmHg or more

New hypertension – Hypertension at or after 20 weeks' gestation in a woman with a diastolic blood pressure of less than 90 mmHg before 20 weeks

New proteinuria – The presence of proteinuria as shown by 1+ (0.3 g/L) or more on proteinuria dipstick testing, a protein:creatinine ratio (PCR) of 30 mg/mmol or more on a random sample, or a urine protein excretion of 300 mg or more per 24 hours

Significant proteinuria – Urine protein excretion ≥ 300 mg per 24 hours

Preeclampsia – New hypertension and significant proteinuria at or after 20 weeks of pregnancy, confirmed if it resolves after delivery

Preexisting hypertension – A diastolic blood pressure pre-pregnancy or at booking (before 20 weeks) of 90 mmHg or more

Superimposed preeclampsia – The development of features of preeclampsia in the context of preexisting hypertension, preexisting proteinuria or both

Fetal compromise (clinical suspicion) – Reduced fetal movements or a small for gestational age fetus.

■ Assessment of risk factors early in pregnancy

Any pregnant woman may develop preeclampsia. Although there are currently no early reliable markers of the condition (reviewed in detail in Chapter 4), the following factors that can be identified early in pregnancy increase the likelihood of preeclampsia developing in any given pregnancy [5]. The presence of any one of these factors should be identified early in pregnancy:

- First pregnancy
- Preeclampsia in any previous pregnancy
- Ten years or more since last baby
- Age 40 years or more
- Body mass index (BMI) of 35 kg/m^2 or more
- Family history of preeclampsia (in mother or sister)
- Booking diastolic blood pressure of 80 mmHg or more
- Booking proteinuria (of $\geq 1+$ on more than one occasion or quantified at ≥ 0.3 g/24 h)

- Multiple pregnancy
- Certain underlying medical conditions:
  - Preexisting hypertension
  - Preexisting renal disease
  - Preexisting diabetes
  - Antiphospholipid antibodies.

Early referral for specialist input to care

Some of these predisposing factors indicate an underlying pathology, concomitant condition, or otherwise high level of obstetric risk related to preeclampsia, which would benefit from specialist input. This may be for further specialist investigation, for clarification of risk, or to advise on early intervention or pharmacological treatment. Pregnant women with one of these predisposing factors for preeclampsia should be offered referral early in pregnancy for specialist input to their antenatal care plan.

Factors which should prompt referral in early pregnancy for specialist input are:
- Multiple pregnancy
- Preeclampsia in any previous pregnancy
- Underlying medical conditions
  - Preexisting hypertension or booking diastolic BP ≥ 90 mmHg
  - Preexisting renal disease or booking proteinuria ($\geq 1+$ on more than one occasion or quantified at ≥ 0.3 g protein/24 h)
  - Preexisting diabetes
  - Antiphospholipid antibodies
- Any two of the following factors: first pregnancy, age 40 years or more, BMI ≥ 35, family history, booking diastolic BP ≥ 80 mmHg < 90 mmHg.

Subsequent obstetric care should be determined on an individual basis. Women should be deemed to be at higher risk and should not be assessed following a schedule of routine care designed for healthy pregnant women with no known risk factors. All pregnant women benefit from a continuity of care and need midwifery care, whatever their obstetric risk; this should be respected, and incorporated into the care plan.

◾ Diagnosis of preeclampsia

Pregnant women, other than those who have received specialist input, should be offered one of two levels of monitoring after 20 weeks for assessment of signs of preeclampsia, according to their level of risk. In the UK this would usually be midwife/primary care physician led in the community.

LEVEL 1 (Routine care): Women with none of the predisposing factors listed above should have preeclampsia assessments at the locally recommended schedule in pregnancy. For healthy parous women with a singleton pregnancy in the UK this is currently at 28, 34, 36, 38, 40, and 41 weeks [6].

LEVEL 2: Women with one predisposing factor listed above and no factor that requires specialist input in early pregnancy should have a regular preeclampsia assessment:

- Between 24 and 32 weeks' gestation, at no more than 3-week intervals, adjusted to individual needs and changes during pregnancy
- Between 32 weeks' gestation and birth, at no more than 2-week intervals, adjusted to individual needs and changes during pregnancy.

Given that preeclampsia can progress to a life-threatening situation on average in two weeks from diagnosis [7], all pregnant women should be advised that preeclampsia can develop between antenatal assessments. They should be made aware of symptoms (see below) and know how to contact their healthcare professional(s) at all times. They should be encouraged to self-refer. Information leaflets for women and their families, and text on CD-ROM in 22 languages may be obtained from Action on Pre-eclampsia (www.apec.org.uk).

At every preeclampsia assessment, the healthcare provider and pregnant women should identify the presence of any one of the five significant signs and symptoms of the onset of preeclampsia:

- New hypertension [8]
- New and/or significant proteinuria [9]
- Maternal symptoms of headache and/or visual disturbance
- Epigastric pain and/or vomiting [10,11]
- Reduced fetal movements [12], small-for-gestational-age (SGA) fetus.

Description of symptoms

- Headache and visual disturbances: severe pounding headache, partial loss of visual acuity, bright/flashing visual disturbances. Migraines can continue during pregnancy and any migraine can be excruciating without being life threatening or associated with signs of preeclampsia.

- Epigastric pain, especially if severe or associated with vomiting. The most sinister epigastric pain is described by the sufferer as severe and is associated with definite tenderness to deep epigastric palpation (the woman winces).

Ensuring accurate blood pressure measurement

The use of inadequate equipment has been identified as part of the substandard care in maternal deaths related to preeclampsia [13]. To reduce errors the following steps should be taken:

- Use accurate calibrated equipment (mercury sphygmomanometer or validated alternative method).
- Use sitting or semi-reclining position so that the arm to be used is at the level of the heart.
- Do not take the blood pressure in the upper arm with the woman laying on her side as this will give falsely lowered readings.
- Use appropriate size of cuff: standard size (13 × 23 cm) for an arm circumference of up to 33 cm, a large size (33 × 15 cm) for an arm circumference between 33 and 41 cm and a thigh cuff (18 × 36 cm) for an arm circumference of 41 cm or more. There is less error introduced by using too large a cuff than by too small a cuff.
- Deflate the cuff slowly, at a rate of 2 mmHg to 3 mmHg per second, taking at least 30 seconds to complete the whole deflation.
- Use Korotkoff V (disappearance of heart sounds) for measurement of diastolic pressure, as this is subject to less intra-observer and inter-observer variation than Korotkoff IV (muffling of heart sounds) and seems to correlate best with intra-arterial pressure in pregnancy. In the 15% of pregnant women whose diastolic pressure falls to zero before the last sound is heard, then both phase IV and phase V readings should be recorded (e.g., 148/84/0 mmHg).
- Measure to the nearest 2 mmHg to avoid digit preference.
- Obtain an estimated systolic pressure by palpation, to avoid an auscultatory gap.

Improving reliability of proteinuria estimate using dipstick testing

Protein dipsticks should be used to estimate proteinuria. The performance of a semiquantitative dipstick is dependent on many variables, including how the dipstick is read (by all comers to a clinic, staff at a routine clinic, trained research observers, or a machine) and the urine concentration of the sample. The performance of quantitative methods of measuring protein is also dependent on a number of factors, such as the adequate collection of a 24-hour sample and the method used to measure protein [14].

In a community setting:

- Reduce false positive results by training the reader of the dipstick to use the correct methodology to read the dipstick tests. Manufacturer's recommendations should be followed.
- The use of automated dipstick readers reduces reader error.
- Do not repeat a test on a second sample as this does not improve the predictive value for significant proteinuria.
- When required, confirm a 1+ result from a dipstick test for proteinuria by measuring protein excretion in a 24-hour urine collection.

■ Management of preeclampsia

Thresholds for further action

(a) **Arrange immediate admission for women with:**
- Diastolic BP ≥ 110 mmHg and new proteinuria $\geq 1+$ on dipstick
- Systolic BP ≥ 170 mmHg and new proteinuria $\geq 1+$ on dipstick
- Diastolic BP ≥ 90 mmHg and new proteinuria $\geq 1+$ on dipstick and significant symptoms.

Box 8.1 Significant symptoms

Epigastric pain, vomiting, headache, visual disturbances, reduced fetal movements, small-for-gestational-age fetus

---

(b) **Refer women for same day hospital step-up assessment with:**
- Diastolic BP ≥ 90 and < 100 mmHg with significant symptoms
- Systolic BP ≥ 160 mmHg (no proteinuria, no symptoms)
- Diastolic BP ≥ 100 mmHg (no proteinuria, no symptoms)
- Diastolic BP ≥ 90 mmHg and new proteinuria $\geq 1+$ on dipstick
- $\geq 1+$ proteinuria on dipstick with significant symptoms
- Epigastric pain with diastolic BP less than 90 mmHg and a trace or no protein.

(c) **Refer women for hospital step-up assessment within 48 hours with:**
  - Diastolic BP ≥ 90 and < 100 mmHg (no proteinuria, no symptoms)
  - 2+ or more on dipstick (no hypertension, no symptoms).

(d) **Repeat preeclampsia assessment within 1 week:**
  - 1+ proteinuria on dipstick (no hypertension, no symptoms).

(e) **Follow local protocols for investigation of fetal compromise or headache.**

Symptoms of fetal compromise may be the first indication of preeclampsia. Consider reducing the interval before next full preeclampsia assessment for women with:

- Headache and or visual disturbances with diastolic blood pressure less than 90 mmHg and a trace of or no proteinuria.
- Reduced movements or SGA fetus with diastolic blood pressure less than 90 mmHg and a trace or no protein. Follow local protocols for investigation of fetal compromise.

See www.apec.org.uk for clinical illustrations of these recommendations.

Hospital step-up assessment

One in ten pregnant women will be referred for developing signs and symptoms (73 000 per year in the UK); around 20% of women progress to preeclampsia [15]. These recommendations are a three-step midwifery assessment of women with suspected preeclampsia referred for a hospital assessment. In the UK, 75% of assessments of women with suspected onset of preeclampsia are in a hospital-based midwifery day assessment unit (DAU).

(i) **For any women with suspected preeclampsia, step 1 assessments are as follows:**
  - Record average blood pressure
  - Estimate proteinuria by dipstick
  - Assess fetal size and well-being
  - Identify maternal symptoms related to preeclampsia.

In the DAU setting, three blood pressure recordings should be taken at least 10 minutes apart. If the first two readings are both less than 140 mmHg systolic and 90 mmHg diastolic, the third reading can be omitted. From these multiple readings, the average systolic and diastolic values can be calculated. The recommendations for minimizing error in blood pressure measurement should be followed. In addition, in the hospital setting, only

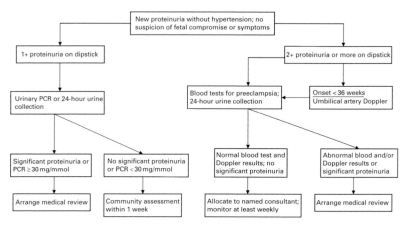

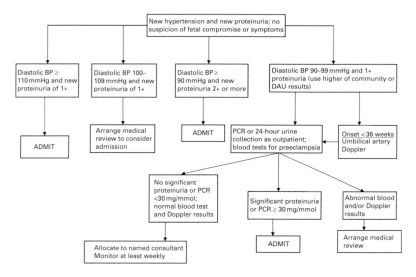

Key: PCR: Urinary protein:creatinine ratio; Blood tests for preeclampsia: platelet count; AST or ALT; serum creatinine; serum urate

Figure 8.1 Flowcharts to describe the identification and subsequent management of women suspected to have preeclampsia or gestational hypertension.

equipment that measures blood pressure accurately in hypertensive pregnant individuals should be used; the use of inaccurate equipment has been implicated in maternal deaths and deaths related to intracerebral hemorrhage have continued to rise. Automated devices that are accurate

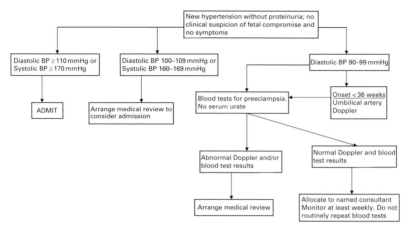

Key: PCR: Urinary protein:creatinine ratio; Blood tests for preeclampsia: platelet count; AST or ALT; serum creatinine; serum urate

Figure 8.1 (*cont.*)

in normotensive women can significantly underestimate blood pressure in women with preeclampsia.

The most accurate non-invasive method for measuring blood pressure is the standard mercury sphygmomanometer. Otherwise, auscultation with alternative pressure gauges should incorporate an aneroid device (calibrated at least every 12 months) or an automated device that has been assessed by protocol for accuracy and validated for use in pregnancy and preeclampsia.

Protein dipsticks should be used to estimate proteinuria. Accuracy is not increased by repeating the test on a new sample. Guidance for improving reliability should be followed.

(ii) For women with confirmed new hypertension or new proteinuria in isolation, step 2 assessments are as follows:

Women may be admitted (with or without the need for medical review), undergo blood tests, umbilical artery Doppler assessments, and/or confirmation of new proteinuria. Unless admitted after these test results, subsequent monitoring will be either from the DAU or in the community (Figure 8.1).

Women with maternal symptoms relating to preeclampsia and/or any clinical suspicion of fetal compromise are not included in the following recommendations. (For evidence-based guidance on investigation of fetal compromise, see national guidelines.) Women should be admitted,

Table 8.1 Pregnancy specific ranges for serum uric acid by gestational age (μmol/L): mean ± 2 standard deviations (SD)

Week	Non-pregnant	4w	8w	12w	16w	24w	32w	36w	38w	Post-partum
mean ± 2SD (μmol/L)	364		328	330	267	285	276	322	344	381	389

Source: From: Lind T, Godfrey KA, Otun H, Philips PR. Changes in serum uric acid concentrations during normal pregnancy. *Br J Obstet Gynaecol* 1984; **91**(2):128–32 [21].

or have a medical review, depending on individual circumstances and following local protocols.

ADMIT women with:

- Diastolic BP ≥ 110 mmHg or systolic BP ≥ 170 mmHg (no proteinuria)
- Diastolic BP ≥ 90 mmHg and new proteinuria ≥ 2+ on dipstick
- Diastolic BP 90–99 mmHg and 1+ proteinuria after step 1: PCR ≥ 30 or significant proteinuria after step 2
- Diastolic BP ≥ 110 mmHg with new proteinuria of 1+.

Arrange medical review to consider admission for women with:

- Diastolic BP 100–109 mmHg or systolic BP 160–169 mmHg (no proteinuria)
- Diastolic BP 100–109 mmHg with new proteinuria of 1+.

Arrange blood tests relating to preeclampsia for women with:

- Diastolic BP 90–99 mmHg and no proteinuria (serum uric acid not required)
- Diastolic BP 90–99 mmHg and 1+ proteinuria (use higher of community or *DAU* dipstick results)
- 2+ or more on dipstick (without new hypertension).

The blood tests relating to preeclampsia are platelet count, transaminases (aspartate transaminase [AST] or alanine transaminase [ALT] as per local availability), serum uric acid, and serum creatinine [10,16–20]; gestational age-specific ranges for AST, ALT, and uric acid are shown in Tables 8.1 and 8.2. A full blood count should be requested. Serum uric acid is not required if there is no proteinuria. Blood tests do not predict the development of preeclampsia in women with new hypertension, but they do identify end-organ damage which can precede both hypertension and proteinuria. In women with new proteinuria (without

Table 8.2 Liver function tests: gestation specific 95% reference ranges (2.5th centile – 97.5th centile) in normal population

	Non-pregnancy	First trimester	Second trimester	Third trimester
AST (iu/L)	7–40	10–28	11–29	11–30
ALT (iu/L)	0–40	6–32	6–32	6–32

Note: Platelet count $< 150 \times 10^{9}$/L.

Creatinine ≥ 90 µmol/L.

Source: From: Girling JC, Dow E, Smith JH. Liver Function tests in pre-eclampsia: importance of comparison with a reference range derived for normal pregnancy. *Br J Obstet Gynaecol* 1997;**104**(2):246–50 [22].

hypertension), abnormal serum uric acid values are associated with abnormal serum creatinine values and poor fetal outcomes. Pregnancy-specific normal ranges for platelets, transaminases, and creatinine should be used, and gestational age-dependent ranges for serum uric acid [21–24].

Arrange umbilical artery Doppler assessment (if onset ≤ 36 completed weeks) for women with:
- Diastolic BP 90–99 mmHg (no proteinuria)
- Diastolic BP 90–99 mmHg and 1+ proteinuria (use higher of community or *DAU* dipstick results)
- 2+ or more on dipstick (no new hypertension).

Evidence advocates the umbilical artery Doppler assessment as the best test for predicting an at-risk fetus in a women with preterm new hypertension [25]. An abnormal umbilical artery Doppler is normally defined as pulsatility index (PI) > 2 standard deviations above the mean and absent or reversed end diastolic flow. Local management protocols should be followed in response to Doppler results. The assessment of women with clinical suspicion of a SGA fetus is not included within this recommendation.

Arrange a urinary protein:creatinine ratio (PCR) or 24-hour urine collection for women with:
- Diastolic BP 90–99 mmHg and 1+ proteinuria (use higher of community or *DAU* dipstick results)
- 1+ proteinuria on dipstick testing (no new hypertension).

Arrange a 24-hour urine collection for women with:
- 2+ or more proteinuria on dipstick testing (no new hypertension).

A laboratory urinary *PCR* from a random sample of less than 30 mg/mmol excludes significant proteinuria and reduces concentration-related errors [26]. A *PCR* > 30 mg/mmol does not reliably confirm or quantify proteinuria. The use of a protein:creatinine ratio instead of a 24-hour urinary protein requires local confirmation of performance, as the method of measuring proteinuria has been shown to modify the results. A 24-hour urine collection should be used to quantify excreted protein. A 24-hour urine collection of ≥ 300 mg/24 h both confirms and quantifies proteinuria.

For women with new hypertension between 90 and 99 mmHg and 1+ proteinuria, the decision to admit should be deferred until the results of the *PCR* are known. This is appropriate only when there are no maternal symptoms or clinical suspicion of fetal compromise.

(iii) Step 3 actions are as follows:

Instigate medical review to clarify management for women with:

- Abnormal blood test and/or Doppler results after step 2
- 1+ or 2+ proteinuria on dipstick testing, no hypertension at step 1; *PCR* ≥ 30 mg/mmol or significant proteinuria at step 2.

Arrange a medical review within the DAU by an experienced clinician (Specialist obstetric doctor) to clarify management.

Allocate to a named consultant

All women who have qualified for a step-up midwifery assessment are at higher risk of preeclampsia and poor outcomes associated with it. With the exception of women who at step 1 assessment have no hypertension, no proteinuria, no relevant symptoms or fetal compromise, we recommend that all women are allocated to a named consultant.

Plan further DAU monitoring for women with:

- Diastolic BP 90–99 mmHg with or without 1+ proteinuria from step 1: *PCR* < 30 mg/mmol or no significant proteinuria and normal blood and Doppler results
- 2+ proteinuria from step 1: *PCR* < 30 mg/mmol or no significant proteinuria and normal blood and Doppler results.

Asymptomatic women with new hypertension (90–99 mmHg), normal blood results, a normal umbilical artery Doppler, and no suspicion of fetal compromise should be invited to undergo follow-up assessment no longer than seven days (minimum standard) after the initial assessment and sooner if appropriate. The frequency of assessment should be agreed with a revised antenatal care plan incorporating input from the named consultant, on an individual basis. Medical review and/or admission should be instigated if there is a change in blood parameters, new symptoms, or a change in signs. If there are no changes in step 1 assessments, repeat blood tests should not be routine. The criteria for admission and medical review in follow-up appointments are the same as for the first step 1 assessment.

Community monitoring should be stepped-up for women with:

- 1+ on dipstick at step 1; *PCR* < 30 mg/mmol or no significant proteinuria. Local protocols to exclude infection should be followed
- Diastolic BP < 90 mmHg, and no proteinuria on dipstick in DAU.

The community lead should be contacted and advised that a woman without confirmed signs or symptoms needs to be assessed in the community within no more than seven days of leaving the DAU. In the subsequent plan of care there should be no more than two weeks between assessments if there is no change in clinical status. Women with transient hypertension or proteinuria are at higher risk of developing preeclampsia (51% will develop hypertension or preeclampsia at final diagnosis) and should no longer be assessed under routine antenatal care. Women with recurrent signs/symptoms will require referral back to the DAU. The criteria to detect and act on any new signs and symptoms are the same.

■ Involvement of women in effective antenatal care

Parents have a full and equal right to determine and be involved in their antenatal care. Therefore they need the opportunity to understand the relevance, to themselves and their babies, of any changes to their antenatal care. The first step-up assessment is the best opportunity to begin this. Women should be offered written and verbal information and sufficient time so that they understand the content and purpose of the DAU assessment and their role in effective antenatal care.

Before a pregnant woman leaves her initial DAU assessment she should have:

- Information to understand the signs and symptoms of fulminating preeclampsia, the rate at which it may develop, and the potential seriousness of her situation
- A mechanism to report and act on any new symptoms that she may notice herself; she should be encouraged to self-monitor

- Handheld notes or a DAU summary from her assessment
- A follow-up appointment
- Allocation to a named consultant
- An agreed mechanism by which she will be informed of any test results and discuss any change to her antenatal care plan within 24 hours
- An understanding that she can be proactive in following up any results and arranging a follow-up appointment if the contact arrangements do not work.

■ Incorporation of these recommendations into local policy and practice

This chapter is based upon the Pre-eclampsia Community Guideline published as a community-based and hospital-based guideline in the *BMJ*, respectively, in 2005 and 2009. The full PRECOG guideline, including all supporting graded evidence, is available at www.apec.org.uk/guidelines.htm.

Under the auspices of the charity Action on Pre-eclampsia there is an active implementation process within the UK with the primary aim of supporting the incorporation of these recommendations into local antenatal care schedules, at the Trust level. Recommended minimum standards for a consultant-led hospital-based maternity DAU providing rapid assessment, investigation, referral, and inpatient treatment are provided. The guideline is available as part of a package, accessed by email, CD-ROM (Word documents for cut/paste or pdf files for printing) or hard copy. The package includes:

- Adoption, training, and implementation flowcharts
- Resource implication audit tool
- The guideline with supporting graded evidence and summary evidence tables
- Slide resource kit for presentation and training
- User aids including stickers, A4 laminated care cards, woman information leaflets
- Audit form and audit support sheet.

There is a central contact-line for information (Action on Preeclampsia email ceo@apec.org.uk or info@apec.org.uk or visit www.apec.org.uk).

1. Waterstone M, Bewley S, Wolfe C. Incidence and predictors of severe obstetric morbidity: case-control study. *BMJ* 2001 May 5;**322**(7294):1089–93; discussion 93–4.

2. Confidential Enquiry into Maternal and Child Health. *Why Mothers Die 1997– 1999*. The Fifth Report of the Confidential Enquiries into Maternal Deaths in the United Kingdom. London, Royal College of Obstetricians and Gynaecologists, 2001.

3. Milne F, Redman C, Walker J, *et al.* Assessing the onset of pre-eclampsia in the hospital day unit: summary of the pre-eclampsia guideline (PRECOG II). *BMJ* 2009;**339**:b3129.

4. Milne F, Redman C, Walker J, *et al.* The pre-eclampsia community guideline (PRECOG): how to screen for and detect onset of pre-eclampsia in the community. *BMJ* 2005;**330**(7491):576–80.

5. Duckitt K, Harrington D. Risk factors for pre-eclampsia at antenatal booking: systematic review of controlled studies. *BMJ* 2005;**330**(7491):565.

6. National Collaboration Centre for Women's and Children's Health. *Antenatal Care: Routine Care for the Healthy Pregnant Woman*. London, RCOG Press, 2008.

7. Sibai BM, Mercer BM, Schiff E, Friedman SA. Aggressive versus expectant management of severe preeclampsia at 28 to 32 weeks' gestation: a randomized controlled trial. *Am J Obstet Gynecol* 1994;**171**(3):818–22.

8. Barton JR, O'Brien JM, Bergauer NK, Jacques DL, Sibai BM. Mild gestational hypertension remote from term: progression and outcome. *Am J Obstet Gynecol* 2001;**184**(5):979–83.

9. Stettler RW, Cunningham FG. Natural history of chronic proteinuria complicating pregnancy. *Am J Obstet Gynecol* 1992;**167**(5):1219–24.

10. Martin JN, Jr., May WL, Magann EF, *et al.* Early risk assessment of severe preeclampsia: admission battery of symptoms and laboratory tests to predict likelihood of subsequent significant maternal morbidity. *Am J Obstet Gynecol* 1999;**180**(6 Pt 1):1407–14.

11. Witlin AG, Saade GR, Mattar F, Sibai BM. Risk factors for abruptio placentae and eclampsia: analysis of 445 consecutively managed women with severe preeclampsia and eclampsia. *Am J Obstet Gynecol* 1999;**180**(6 Pt 1):1322–9.

12. Simon A, Ohel G, Mor-Yosef S, Brjejinski A, Sadovsky E. Fetal movements in hypertensive pregnancies. *Aust N Z J Obstet Gynaecol* 1985;**25**(3):179–81.

13. Lewis GE. (ed.) The Confidential Enquiry into Maternal and Child Health. *Saving Mother's Lives: reviewing maternal deaths to make motherhood safer – 2003–2005*. The Seventh Report on Confidential Enquiries into Maternal Deaths in the United Kingdom. London, CEMACH, 2007.

14. Durnwald C, Mercer B. A prospective comparison of total protein/creatinine ratio versus 24-hour urine protein in women with suspected preeclampsia. *Am J Obstet Gynecol* 2003;**189**(3):848–52.

15. Anumba DOC, Lincoln K, Robson S. Predictive value of clinical and laboratory indices at first assessment in women referred with suspected gestational hypertension. *Hypertens Pregnancy* 2010;**29**(2):163–79.

16. Bailey DJ, Walton SM. Routine investigations might be useful in pre-eclampsia, but not in gestational hypertension. *Aust N Z J Obstet Gynaecol* 2005;**45**(2):144–7.

17. Calvert SM, Tuffnell DJ, Haley J. Poor predictive value of platelet count, mean platelet volume and serum urate in hypertension in pregnancy. *Eur J Obstet Gynecol Reprod Biol* 1996;**64**(2):179–84.

18. Hauth JC, Ewell MG, Levine RJ, *et al.* Pregnancy outcomes in healthy nulliparas who developed hypertension. Calcium for Preeclampsia Prevention Study Group. *Obstet Gynecol* 2000;**95**(1):24–8.

19. Roberts JM, Bodnar LM, Lain KY, *et al.* Uric acid is as important as proteinuria in identifying fetal risk in women with gestational hypertension. *Hypertension* 2005;**46**(6):1263–9.

20. Paternoster DM, Stella A, Mussap M, *et al.* Predictive markers of pre-eclampsia in hypertensive disorders of pregnancy. *Int J Gynaecol Obstet* 1999;**66**(3):237–43.

21. Lind T, Godfrey KA, Otun H, Philips PR. Changes in serum uric acid concentrations during normal pregnancy. *Br J Obstet Gynaecol* 1984;**91**(2):128–32.

22. Girling JC, Dow E, Smith JH. Liver function tests in pre-eclampsia: importance of comparison with a reference range derived for normal pregnancy. *Br J Obstet Gynaecol* 1997;**104**(2):246–50.

23. Tygart SG, McRoyan DK, Spinnato JA, McRoyan CJ, Kitay DZ. Longitudinal study of platelet indices during normal pregnancy. *Am J Obstet Gynecol* 1986;**154**(4):883–7.

24. Girling JC. Re-evaluation of plasma creatinine concentration in normal pregnancy. *J Obstet Gynaecol* 2000;**20**(2):128–31.

25. Neilson JP, Alfirevic Z. Doppler ultrasound for fetal assessment in high risk pregnancies. *Cochrane Database Syst Rev (Online)* 2000;(2):CD000073.

26. Papanna R, Mann LK, Kouides RW, Glantz JC. Protein/creatinine ratio in preeclampsia: a systematic review. *Obstet Gynecol* 2008;**112**(1):135–44.

FURTHER READING

Milne F, Redman C, Walker J, *et al.* The pre-eclampsia community guideline (PRECOG): how to screen for and detect onset of pre-eclampsia in the community *BMJ* 2005;**330**:576–80.

Milne F, Redman C, Walker J, *et al.* Assessing the onset of pre-eclampsia in the hospital day unit: summary of the pre-eclampsia guideline (PRECOG II) *BMJ* 2009;**339**:b3129.

National Institute for Health and Clinical Excellence (NICE). *Clinical Guideline 6: Antenatal Care: Routine Care for Healthy Pregnant Women,* 2003. www.nice.org.uk.

National Institute for Health and Clinical Excellence (NICE). *Clinical Guideline on Hypertensive Disorders During Pregnancy,* 2010. www.nice.org.uk.

Management of severe preeclampsia

9

Baha M. Sibai and Errol R. Norwitz

■ Introduction

Preeclampsia is a multisystem disorder that is unique to human pregnancy. The clinical findings of preeclampsia can manifest primarily as a maternal syndrome that is characterized by hypertension and proteinuria with or without other symptoms and abnormal laboratory tests, or as a fetal syndrome that is characterized by fetal growth restriction, reduced amniotic fluid, or abnormal fetal oxygenation [1]. Consequently, preeclampsia is associated with substantial maternal and perinatal morbidity and mortality worldwide, particularly in developing countries [1,2]. Maternal and perinatal prognosis depends on the presence or absence of factors listed in Table 9.1. In general, maternal and perinatal outcomes are usually favorable in healthy nulliparous women who develop mild preeclampsia beyond 36 weeks' gestation, whereas the outcomes are less favorable in those having any of the factors listed in Table 9.1.

Preeclampsia is usually classified as either "mild" or "severe" based on the severity of maternal blood pressure elevation, amount of proteinuria, and presence or absence of organ dysfunction [1,3,4]. Preeclampsia is considered "severe" when there is new-onset hypertension plus proteinuria after 20 weeks' gestation in association with any of the factors listed in Table 9.2 [4].

■ Incidence and severity of preeclampsia

The reported incidence of preeclampsia ranges from 2% to 7% of all pregnancies [1]. The incidence depends on parity, maternal age, body

Hypertension in Pregnancy, ed. Alexander Heazell, Errol R. Norwitz, Louise C. Kenny, and Philip N. Baker. Published by Cambridge University Press. © Cambridge University Press 2010.

Table 9.1 Factors associated with adverse maternal and perinatal outcome in women with preeclampsia

- Severe preeclampsia
  - Severe hypertension with cerebral symptoms (headache, visual aberrations)
  - Severe epigastric/abdominal pain and elevated liver enzymes
  - Severe thrombocytopenia with evidence of bleeding (such as mucosal bleeding)
- Gestational age at time of diagnosis
  - < 28 weeks (associated with poor outcome for mother and fetus)
  - 28–32 weeks (associated with increased neonatal morbidity)
- Presence of fetal syndrome
  - Fetal growth restriction
  - Oligohydramnios
  - Abnormal umbilical artery Doppler velocimetry studies
- Presence of preexisting medical conditions
  - Chronic hypertension or renal disease
  - Connective tissue disease
  - Pre-gestational diabetes mellitus
  - Obesity
- Multiple pregnancy
- Quality of medical, obstetric, and neonatal care

Table 9.2 Criteria for the diagnosis of severe preeclampsia

Criteria	Definition
Symptoms	
• Symptoms of central nervous system dysfunction	Subjective complaints of blurred vision, scotomata, altered mental status, and/or severe headache
• Symptoms of liver capsule distention or rupture	Subjective complaints of persistent right upper-quadrant and/or epigastric pain
Signs	
• Blood pressure criteria	Sitting blood pressure $\geq$ 160 mmHg systolic and/or $\geq$ 110 mmHg diastolic on 2 separate occasions at rest at least 6 hours apart
• Eclampsia	Generalized seizures and/or unexplained coma in the setting of preeclampsia and in the absence of other neurological conditions
• Pulmonary edema or cyanosis	Excessive fluid accumulation in the lungs
• Cerebrovascular accident (stroke)	Acute loss of brain function (as evidenced by focal neurological signs, altered mental status, and/or coma) because of a disturbance in the vasculature that supplies blood to the brain

Table 9.2 (*cont.*)

Criteria	Definition
• Cortical blindness	Partial or total loss of vision in a normal-appearing eye that is caused by damage to the visual region of the occipital cortex
• FGR	Estimated fetal weight < 5th percentile for gestational age or < 10th percentile for gestational age with evidence of fetal compromise (oligohydramnios, abnormal umbilical artery Doppler velocimetry)
Laboratory findings	
• Proteinuria	> 5 g per 24 hours or $\geq 3+$ on 2 random urine samples that are collected at least 4 hours apart
• Oliguria and/or renal failure	Urine output < 500 mL per 24 hours and/or serum creatinine > 1.2 mg/dL
• HELLP syndrome	Evidence of hemolysis (abnormal peripheral smear, total bilirubin > 1.2 mg/dL, lactate dehydrogenase > 600 U/L), elevated liver enzymes (alanine aminotransferase > 70 U/L, lactate dehydrogenase > 600 U/L), and low platelets ($< 100\,000$ platelets/mm^3)
• Hepatocellular injury	Serum transaminase levels $\geq 2 \times$ normal
• Thrombocytopenia	$< 100\,000$ platelets/mm^3
• Coagulopathy	Prolonged prothrombin time (> 1.4 seconds), low platelet count ($< 100\,000$ platelets/mm^3), and low fibrinogen (< 300 mg/dL)

Note: HELLP, hemolysis, elevated liver enzymes, and low platelets.
Source: From: Norwitz ER, Funai EF. Expectant management of severe preeclampsia remote from term: hope for the best, but expect the worst. *Am J Obstet Gynecol* 2008;**199**:209–12[4].

mass index, number of fetuses, and presence or absence of preexisting medical conditions [1,2,5]. In clinical practice, most cases of preeclampsia are mild and occur at term in healthy nulliparous women [1,2,5].

The incidence of severe preeclampsia ranges from 0.6% to 1.2% of pregnancies in western countries [5–7]. Preterm preeclampsia (< 37 weeks) develops in 0.6% to 1.5% of all pregnancies, and severe and early-onset preeclampsia (< 34 weeks) develop in 0.3% of pregnancies [5,8]. The reported incidence of severe and/or early-onset preeclampsia is substantially higher in women with previous history of preeclampsia, in those with long-standing diabetes mellitus, chronic hypertension, morbid obesity, thrombophilia, and in those with multi-fetal gestations [1,5,9–11].

Table 9.3 Maternal and perinatal complications in severe preeclampsia

Maternal complications	• HELLP syndrome with or without liver hemorrhage
	• Placental abruption with or without disseminated intravascular coagulopathy (DIC)
	• Pulmonary edema
	• Acute renal failure (which may require dialysis)
	• Eclampsia (which may be complicated by aspiration pneumonitis)
	• Retinal detachment with or without underlying retinopathy
	• Adult respiratory distress syndrome
	• Stoke (encephalopathy or cerebral hemorrhage)
	• Death
	• Long-term cardiovascular and renal morbidity
Fetal complications	• Fetal growth restriction
	• Oligohydramnios
	• Hypoxia-acidosis
	• Preterm delivery
	• Death
	• Long-term morbidity
	– Neurological deficit
	– Cerebral palsy
	– Cardiovascular disease

■ Maternal and perinatal outcome

Pregnancies complicated by severe preeclampsia – particularly those remote from term – are associated with serious maternal and perinatal complications. Maternal and perinatal complications may be either acute or long term (Table 9.3) [1,6,12,13]. Maternal long-term morbidity may be related to the acute complications (such as renal failure, stroke, or retinal injury) and to the fact that some of these women have preexisting factors for increased risk of cardiovascular complications later in life [12,13]. In addition, infant complications may be related to chronic or acute hypoxia and/or to prematurity and fetal growth restriction.

■ Management of severe preeclampsia

The clinical course of severe preeclampsia is usually characterized by progressive deterioration in both maternal and fetal conditions [14]. As a result, traditional management has focused on maternal safety by means of expedited delivery, which is the ultimate and only effective cure for preeclampsia. Although delivery is always appropriate for the mother, it might not be best for a very premature fetus. Currently, there is general agreement that patients with severe preeclampsia should be delivered if the disease develops at ≥ 34 weeks of gestation [14]. The management of patients with severe preeclampsia < 34 weeks is more controversial, and a number of authors have suggested some form of expectant management in an attempt to prolong gestation and improve perinatal outcome. In 2007, Sibai and Barton summarized studies that had been published up to 2006 and proposed guidelines for the expectant management of severe preeclampsia remote from term [14]. In the following sections, we will review the maternal and perinatal risks of the treatment of severe preeclampsia, particularly those remote from term. We will also identify the optimal candidates for such management, the contraindications, as well as indications for immediate delivery. Finally, we will address a number of topics that remain a matter of controversy in expectant management.

Summary of published studies

When one reviews the published literature on expectant management of severe preeclampsia remote from term, it becomes clear that most of the studies are retrospective or observational in nature. There are only two prospective randomized trials addressing this issue [15,16], both of which are underpowered to adequately answer the question of whether such management is safe. There is also one large multicenter trial that compares two methods of management: antihypertensives alone versus antihypertensives plus plasma volume expansion [17]. The trial by Odendaal *et al.* included only 38 patients [15], whereas that reported by Sibai *et al.* included 95 subjects [16]. Both of these trials reported improved perinatal outcome and minimal maternal morbidity with expectant management. The trial reported by Ganzevoort *et al.* included 216 patients [17], and reported no additional benefit from plasma volume expansion during expectant management. It is important to note that this latter study had a heterogeneous group of patients (including severe fetal growth restriction [FGR], thrombocytopenia, HELLP [hemolysis, elevated liver enzymes, and low platelets] syndrome, eclampsia, and chronic hypertension) at the time of enrollment. As a result, the trial reported a high baseline perinatal mortality and morbidity.

Observational and retrospective studies

There are numerous retrospective studies that describe expectant management of severe preeclampsia at 24–34 weeks' gestation [7,10,11,18–26]. These studies included patients with preeclampsia, superimposed preeclampsia, with or without symptoms, with or without FGR at enrollment, and variable criteria to define severe preeclampsia. As a result, the median or average pregnancy prolongation and ranges as well as the perinatal mortality and maternal complications are highly variable among these studies.

In these studies, maternal and/or perinatal complications are the most common indication for delivery during expectant management. Non-reassuring fetal testing is the most common fetal indication with a reported rate of 27% to 74%. The reported perinatal mortality rate in these studies ranged from 0% to 16.6% [14]. This variation in perinatal mortality rate reflects differences in gestational age at inclusion, in the presence or absence of severe FGR and HELLP syndrome, and/or quality of neonatal care (including year of reporting and country of origin). In recent studies conducted in the western countries, the perinatal mortality rate was 0% when expectant management was initiated at ≥ 30 weeks' gestation [7,17,26].

There is also the potential for maternal complications during any protocol for expectant management of severe preeclampsia. Since 1990, there was one maternal death reported among 1790 women who underwent expectant treatment of severe preeclampsia at > 24 weeks' gestation [5,14,26–28]. In contrast, maternal morbidity such as HELLP syndrome (4–25%), placental abruption (4–22%), and pulmonary edema (1–9%) remain high [14].

Management of severe preeclampsia < 25 weeks' gestation

Severe preeclampsia that develops at this early gestational age is associated with a high perinatal mortality and morbidity [14,27–35]. Immediate delivery, on the other hand, is associated with extremely high neonatal mortality and morbidities [31,34]. There are limited data regarding maternal and perinatal outcomes during expectant management in such women. The number of such patients reported in the literature is 190, with perinatal survival rates ranging from 0% at $<23^{+0}$ weeks to approximately 20% at 23^{+0} to 23^{+6} weeks of gestation at the time of expectant management. In contrast, the reported perinatal survival rate at 24^{+0} to 24^{+6} weeks in studies reported from Australia and the United States was 60% to 70% [27]. Overall, there were 31 surviving infants in this group of patients, but detailed long-term neurological outcome data were provided for only a limited number of these infants. In addition, there was one maternal death (0.5%) in this group; the patient had HELLP syndrome and eclampsia and underwent expectant management at 23 weeks of gestation [32]. Moreover, reported maternal morbidities in these studies were very high ranging from 31% to 67% [27]. Thus, expectant management should not be offered to patients with severe preeclampsia below 23 weeks and probably not in women below 24 weeks [14,27]. Extensive counseling by an experienced perinatologist is indicated in such women.

Expectant management in patients with FGR

There are no prospective randomized trials evaluating the risks and benefits of expectant management in such patients. There are only four retrospective or observational studies evaluating expectant management in such women, and only two adequately described the outcome of pregnancies known to have FGR at the onset of expectant management [17,18]. The other two studies only described the outcome of those pregnancies who had FGR at the time of delivery [24,36]. The results of these studies remain inconclusive, but it appears that the presence of severe FGR should be considered a contraindication to expectant management, particularly in pregnancies ≥ 30 weeks' gestation [4].

■ Recommended management of severe preeclampsia

The main objective of the management of severe preeclampsia must always be the safety of both the mother and fetus. As a result, all patients with severe preeclampsia should receive prompt hospitalization on labor and delivery for intensive observation of maternal and fetal well-being [14]. All patients should receive intravenous magnesium sulfate to prevent convulsions (eclampsia) and antihypertensive medications to lower blood pressure if it is severely and dangerously elevated (generally regarded as a systolic pressure ≥ 160 mmHg and/or diastolic pressure ≥ 110 mmHg). The goal of antihypertensive therapy is to keep the systolic blood pressure between 140 and 155 mmHg and diastolic blood pressure between 90 and 105 mmHg. During this initial observation period, the maternal clinical condition, laboratory findings, and fetal gestational age and well-being should be assessed and a decision made regarding the need for immediate delivery. Patients with a gestational age of $< 23^{+0}$ or $\geq 34^{+0}$ weeks, those with non-reassuring fetal testing, and those with severe complications (such as eclampsia, neurological deficit, pulmonary edema, acute renal failure, coagulopathy, and placental abruption) should be delivered once the maternal condition is stable [14]. In addition, expectant management of patients with preeclampsia between 23^{+0} and 23^{+6} is associated with extremely high maternal and perinatal morbidity and mortality rates [27–35]. As such, continued expectant management in such patients should only be considered as an option after extensive counseling by an experienced perinatologist, with particular attention paid to the potential for long-term severe neurological deficits in infants that survive. If the woman elects continued expectant treatment, she should be offered ante-natal corticosteroids for fetal lung maturity; however, she should be informed that there are no reliable data to support their use at this early gestational age. Subsequent management in these patients should be similar to those between 24^{+0} and 33^{+6} weeks of gestation.

Patients with severe preeclampsia between 24^{+0} and 33^{+6} should be given a course of antenatal corticosteroids to accelerate fetal lung maturity, and then managed according to the algorithm described in Figure 9.1. This proposed management is based on review of the available literature and on expert opinion. The management of such patients should be individualized based on their clinical response during the initial 24-hour observation period. If blood pressure is adequately controlled and fetal testing is reassuring, magnesium sulfate seizure prophylaxis can be discontinued and the patient monitored closely on the antepartum high-risk ward until 33^{+6} weeks' gestation is achieved or until she develops another maternal or fetal indication for immediate delivery (Table 9.4). It is important to emphasize that this approach should be practiced in a hospital with adequate maternal and neonatal intensive care facilities. If not available at the admission hospital, the patient should be transferred to a more appropriate facility as soon as the maternal and fetal conditions allow. All patients should be seen and counseled by both anesthesia and

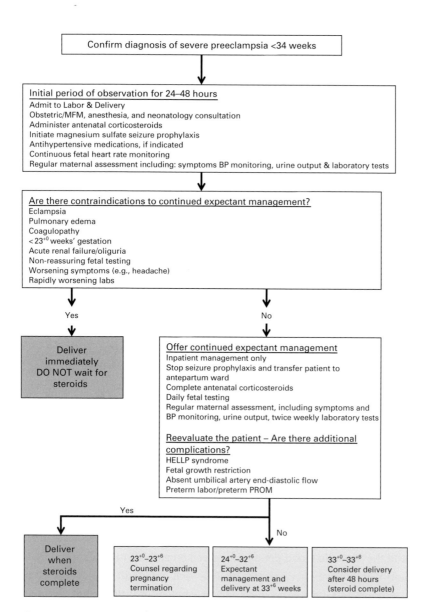

Figure 9.1 Proposed clinical algorithm for the management of severe preeclampsia less than 34 weeks' gestation. MFM, maternal–fetal medicine; PROM, premature rupture of membranes.

neonatology on admission to hospital, because of the potential for an acute event requiring emergent delivery.

Once on the antepartum service, the patient's blood pressure should be measured every 4–6 hours. The standard technique for measuring blood

Table 9.4 Indications for immediate delivery during expectant management of severe preeclampsia

Fetal indications	• ≥ 34 weeks' gestation
	• 33–34 weeks with documented lung maturity or after steroid use
	• Estimated fetal weight < 5th percentile by ultrasound
	• Abnormal fetal testing
	• Repetitive variable or late decelerations
	• Biophysical profile (BPP) ≤ 4 on 2 occasions at least 4 hours apart
	• Persistent severe oligohydramnios (defined as amniotic fluid index < 5 cm or maximum vertical pocket < 2 cm)
	• Persistent reverse end-diastolic flow on umbilical artery Doppler velocimetry
	• Rupture of membranes
Maternal indications	• Preterm labor or vaginal bleeding
	• Eclampsia or encephalopathy
	• Pulmonary edema or renal failure
	• Persistent oliguria despite therapy
	• Persistent thrombocytopenia
	• Severe epigastric pain or cerebral symptoms
	• Maternal request
	• Severe hypertension unresponsive to maximum drug therapy

pressure in pregnancy is for the patient to be in the sitting position at rest for at least 5 minutes using the appropriate size blood pressure cuff and the fifth Korotkoff sounds (disappearance, not muffling) to designate the diastolic pressure. Patients should receive antihypertensive drugs as needed to keep the systolic blood pressure between 140 and 155 mmHg and the diastolic blood pressure between 90 and 105 mmHg. Appropriate antihypertensive medications include oral nifedipine 10–20 mg every 4–6 hours (40–120 mg per day) and/or labetalol 200–800 mg orally every 8 hours (600–2400 mg per day). An alternative regimen may include nifedipine XL 30 mg every 8–12 hours. If the patient develops persistent severe hypertension while her oral antihypertensive regimen is being adjusted, blood pressure measurements should be assessed every 15 minutes. If the blood pressure remains in the severe range after 30–60 minutes, the patient should be transferred immediately to the labor and delivery unit for more intensive monitoring and treatment. She should also receive an acute antihypertensive bolus of either nifedipine 10 mg orally, labetalol 20 mg IV, or hydralazine 5–10 mg IV as needed [14]. Patients with persistent severe hypertension despite maximum doses of antihypertensive agents should be restarted on magnesium sulfate seizure prophylaxis and delivered.

Throughout the period of expectant management, the patient should be evaluated regularly to confirm both maternal and fetal well-being. Maternal assessment should include frequent evaluation of her symptoms (headache, blurred or double vision, confusion, nausea, vomiting, epigastric or upper abdominal pain, shortness of breath, uterine activity, and vaginal bleeding), physical examination (upper abdominal tenderness, tendon reflexes, and clonus), fluid intake and output, and laboratory testing. Serial laboratory testing should be performed at least twice weekly, including full blood count (FBC) with platelet count, serum transaminases, lactate dehydrogenase, and creatinine. Fetal assessment should include daily or twice daily fetal kick counts, at least daily non-stress testing (NST) with uterine activity monitoring, serial biophysical profile (BPP) if the gestational age is early or if the NST is non-reactive, and twice weekly amniotic fluid assessment [14–19,23–27,37]. Severe oligohydramnios is defined as an amniotic fluid index (AFI) < 5 cm or maximum vertical pocket < 2 cm on at least two occasions at least 24 hours apart. In the absence of ruptured membranes, severe oligohydramnios should be considered a contraindication for continued expectant management in all patients with a gestational age beyond 30 weeks irrespective of other fetal test results. In those at or below 30 weeks' gestation, pregnancy may be continued if the NST is reassuring and umbilical artery Doppler velocimetry is normal. Umbilical artery Doppler velocimetry studies should be performed weekly or twice weekly if FGR is suspected or if initial testing reveals abnormal end-diastolic flow [7,11,24,25,38,39]. Umbilical artery Doppler velocimetry studies showing persistent reverse diastolic flow following initial maternal–fetal stabilization should be considered an indication for immediate delivery. Ultrasonographic assessment of fetal growth should be performed every two to three weeks while the patient is on the antepartum service. The absence of interval fetal growth over a two- to three-week period may be an indication for delivery. Other indications for abandoning continued expectant management and proceeding with immediate delivery are summarized in Table 9.4.

Once the decision has been made to proceed with delivery, the patients should be transferred to the labor and delivery unit and started on magnesium sulfate seizure prophylaxis. Such prophylaxis should be continued throughout labor and delivery and for at least 24 hours postpartum.

■ Mode of delivery in patients with severe preeclampsia

There are no randomized trials that compare the optimal mode of delivery in women with severe preeclampsia. All available data are based on retrospective studies [40–44]. In general, the decision of whether to perform a Cesarean delivery or attempt induction of labor should be based on the following factors: gestational age, fetal presentation, presence of labor, cervical status (Bishop score), and fetal testing. On the basis of available data, induction of labor and attempted vaginal delivery is a reasonable option for patients with a gestational age $> 32^{+0}$ weeks, a vertex presentation, and the absence of fetal or medical contraindications. The success rate in this situation is $> 60\%$. In contrast, the Cesarean delivery rate among reported studies in women receiving expectant management at 24–33 weeks' gestation ranges from 66% to 96%, with the higher Cesarean delivery rates for patients with severe preeclampsia < 28 weeks [14]. This observation is not surprising given that the indication for delivery in such women is typically an acute deterioration in either maternal or fetal condition. Thus, a very small percentage of these patients would be appropriate candidates for induction of labor.

For patients undergoing induction of labor for severe preeclampsia at ≥ 37 weeks, the reported Cesarean delivery rate is 28%, whereas it is 32% for those undergoing induction at 34–36 weeks' gestation [43]. For those undergoing induction at 28–32 weeks, the reported Cesarean delivery rate ranged from 45% to 53% [40,43,44]. For those at < 28 weeks, the Cesarean delivery rate was 91–96% [41,42]. Therefore, it is reasonable to recommend elective Cesarean for all patients with severe preeclampsia requiring delivery < 28 weeks and for patients with severe preeclampsia requiring delivery < 32 weeks if there is evidence of FGR, severe oligohydramnios, or reverse umbilical artery end-diastolic flow on Doppler velocimetry.

■ Postpartum management of patients with severe preeclampsia

During the immediate postpartum period, women with severe preeclampsia should receive close monitoring of blood pressure and symptoms, and should have an accurate measurement of all fluid intake and urinary output. Such women typically receive large amounts of intravenous fluids during labor as a result of preloading before epidural analgesia placement, oxytocin administration, and intrapartum and postpartum magnesium sulfate seizure prophylaxis. In addition, the postpartum period in such women is characterized by mobilization of large amounts of extracellular fluid resulting in a significant increase in intravascular volume. As a result, such women are at increased risk for pulmonary edema and exacerbation of severe hypertension in the immediate postpartum period. Once the fetus is delivered, there is no longer a concern about reduced uteroplacental blood flow from lowering the maternal blood pressure. As such, it is reasonable to be more aggressive with blood pressure control. We recommend using antihypertensive medications to maintain the systolic blood pressure ≤ 155 mmHg and the diastolic blood pressure ≤ 105 mmHg. Most authorities would recommend nifedipine (10 mg orally every 4–6 hours) or labetalol (200–400 mg orally every 8–12 hours), although some authors have suggested a short course of oral furosemide (20 mg daily) with potassium supplementation [45].

■ Conclusion

Severe preeclampsia remains a major cause of maternal and perinatal morbidity and mortality. Early diagnosis and aggressive management is required to optimize outcome for both mother and fetus. There is absolutely no benefit to the mother remaining pregnant once a diagnosis of severe preeclampsia is made, but continued expectant management in select patients remote from term may be appropriate with a view to getting the fetus to a more favorable gestational age before delivery and thereby improving perinatal outcome. Such a management strategy should only be undertaken after careful consultation and counseling with an experienced perinatologist, and with patient consent. Moreover, such patients should be closely observed as inpatients in an institution with the capacity to handle potential complications (such as eclampsia, HELLP syndrome, pulmonary edema, or coagulopathy) and to affect immediate delivery, if indicated.

REFERENCES

1. Sibai B, Dekker G, Kupfermic M. Pre-eclampsia. *Lancet* 2005;**365**:785–99.
2. Report of the National High Blood Pressure Education Program. Working group report on high blood pressure in pregnancy. *Am J Obstet Gynecol* 2000;**183**:S1–22.
3. American College of Obstetricians and Gynecologists. Diagnosis and management of pre-eclampsia and eclampsia. ACOG Practice Bulletin No. 33. *Obstet Gynecol* 2002;**99**:159–67.
4. Norwitz ER, Funai EF. Expectant management of severe preeclampsia remote from term: hope for the best, but expect the worst. *Am J Obstet Gynecol* 2008;**199**:209–12.
5. Catov JM, Ness RB, Kip KE, Olsen J. Risk of early or severe pre-eclampsia related to preexisting conditions. *Int J Epidemiol* 2007;**36**:412–19.
6. Zhang J, Meikle S, Trumble A. Severe maternal morbidity associated with hypertensive disorders in pregnancy in the United States. *Hypertens Pregnancy* 2003;**22**:203–12.
7. Haddad B, Deis S, Goffinet F, *et al.* Maternal and perinatal outcomes during expectant management of 239 severe preeclamptic women between 24 and 33 weeks' gestation. *Am J Obstet Gynecol* 2004;**190**:1590–5.
8. Gupta LM, Gaston L, Chauhan SP. Detection of fetal growth restriction with preterm severe pre-eclampsia: experience at two tertiary centers. *Am J Perinatol* 2008;**25**:247–9.
9. Hnat MD, Sibai BM, Caritis S, *et al.* Perinatal outcome in women with recurrent pre-eclampsia compared with women who develop pre-eclampsia as nulliparous. *Am J Obstet Gynecol* 2002;**186**:422–6.
10. Visser W, Wallenburg HCS. Maternal and perinatal outcome of temporizing management in 254 consecutive patients with severe pre-eclampsia remote from term. *Eur J Obstet Gynecol Reprod Biol* 1995;**63**:147–54.
11. Vigil-DeGarcia P, Montufar-Rueda C, Ruiz J. Expectant management of severe pre-eclampsia between 24 and 34 weeks' gestation. *Eur J Obstet Gynecol Reprod Biol* 2003;**107**:24–7.
12. Magnussen EB, Vatlen LJ, Lund-Nilsen TI, *et al.* Pregnancy cardiovascular risk factors as predictors of pre-eclampsia: population based cohort study. *BMJ* 2007;**335**:978–81.
13. Sibai BM. Intergenerational factors: A missing link for pre-eclampsia, fetal growth restriction, and cardiovascular disease? *Hypertension* 2008;**51**:993–4.

14. Sibai BM, Barton JR. Expectant management of severe pre-eclampsia remote from term: patient selection, treatment, and delivery indications. *Am J Obstet Gynecol* 2007;**196**:514.e1–9.

15. Odendaal HJ, Pattinson RC, Bam R, Grove D, Kotze TJ. Aggressive or expectant management for patients with severe pre-eclampsia between 28–34 weeks' gestation: a randomized controlled trial. *Obstet Gynecol* 1990;**76**:1070–5.

16. Sibai BM, Mercer BM, Schiff E, Friedman SA. Aggressive versus expectant management of severe pre-eclampsia at 28 to 32 weeks' gestation: a randomized controlled trial. *Am J Obstet Gynecol* 1994;**171**:818–22.

17. Ganzevoort W, Rep A, Bonsel GJ, *et al.* A randomized controlled trial comparing two temporizing management strategies, one with and one without plasma volume expansion, for severe pre-eclampsia. *BJOG* 2005;**112**:1358–68.

18. Chammas MF, Nguyen TM, Li MA, Nuwayhid BS, Castro LC. Expectant management of severe preterm pre-eclampsia: is intrauterine growth restriction an indication for immediate delivery? *Am J Obstet Gynecol* 2000;**183**:853–8.

19. Sibai BM, Akl S, Fairlie F, Moretti M. A protocol for managing severe pre-eclampsia in the second trimester. *Am J Obstet Gynecol* 1990;**163**:733–8.

20. Chua S, Redman CW. Prognosis for pre-eclampsia complicated by 5 g or more of proteinuria in 24 hours. *Eur J Obstet Gynecol Reprod Biol* 1992;**43**:9–12.

21. Olah KS, Redman WG, Gee H. Management of severe, early pre-eclampsia: is conservative management justified? *Eur J Obstet Gynecol Reprod Biol* 1993;**51**:175–80.

22. Hall DR, Odendaal HJ, Steyn DW, Grove D. Expectant management of early onset, severe pre-eclampsia: maternal outcome. *Br J Obstet Gynaecol* 2000;**107**:1252–7.

23. Hall DR, Odendaal HJ, Kristen GF, Smith J, Grove D. Expectant management of early onset, severe pre-eclampsia: perinatal outcome. *Br J Obstet Gynaecol* 2000;**107**:1258–64.

24. Shear RM, Rinfret D, Leduc L. Should we offer expectant management in cases of severe preterm pre-eclampsia with fetal growth restriction? *Am J Obstet Gynecol* 2005;**192**:1119–25.

25. Oettle C, Hall D, Roux A, Grove D. Early onset severe pre-eclampsia: expectant management at a secondary hospital in close association with a tertiary institution. *BJOG* 2005;**112**:84–8.

26. Bombrys AE, Barton JR, Habli M, Sibai BM. Expectant management of severe pre-eclampsia at $27^{0/7}$–$33^{6/7}$ weeks' gestation: maternal and perinatal outcomes according to gestational age by weeks at onset of expectant management. *Am J Perinatol* 2009;**26**:441–6.

27. Bombrys AE, Barton JR, Nowacki E, Habli M, Sibai BM. Expectant management of severe pre-eclampsia at <27 weeks' gestation: maternal and perinatal outcomes according to gestational age by weeks at onset of expectant management. *Am J Obstet Gynecol* 2008;**199**:247.e1–6.

28. Sezik M, Ozkaya O, Sezik HT, Yapar EG. Expectant management of severe pre-eclampsia presenting before 25 weeks of gestation. *Med Sci Monit* 2007;**13**:523–7.

29. Moodley J, Koranteng SA, Rout C. Expectant management of early onset of severe pre-eclampsia in Durban. *S Afr Med J* 1993;**83**:584–7.

30. Hall DR, Odendaal HJ, Steyn DW. Expectant management of severe pre-eclampsia in the mid-trimester. *Eur J Obstet Gynecol Reprod Biol* 2001;**96**:168–72.

31. Jenkins SM, Head BB, Hauth JC. Severe pre-eclampsia at < 25 weeks of gestation: maternal and neonatal outcomes. *Am J Obstet Gynecol* 2002;**186**:790–5.

32. Gaugler-Senden IP, Huijssoon AG, Visser W, Steegers EAP, deGroot CJM. Maternal and perinatal outcome of pre-eclampsia with onset before 24 weeks' gestation: audit in a tertiary referral center. *Eur J Obstet Gynecol Reprod Biol* 2006;**128**:216–21.

33. Budden A, Wilkinson L, Buksh MJ, McCowan L. Pregnancy outcome in women presenting with pre-eclampsia at less than 25 weeks' gestation. *Aust N Z J Obstet Gynaecol* 2006;**46**:407–12.

34. Hall DR, Grove D, Carstens E. Early-pre-eclampsia: what proportion of women qualify for expectant management and if not, why not? *Eur J Obstet Gynecol Reprod Biol* 2006;**128**:169–74.

35. Withagen MIJ, Wallenburg HCS, Steegers EAP, Hop WCJ, Visser W. Morbidity and development in childhood of infants born after temporising treatment of early onset pre-eclampsia. *BJOG* 2004;**112**:910–14.

36. Haddad B, Kayem G, Deis S, Sibai BM. Are perinatal and maternal outcomes different during expectant management of severe pre-eclampsia in the presence of intrauterine growth restriction? *Am J Obstet Gynecol* 2007;**196**:237.e1–5.

37. Chari RS, Friedman SA, O'Brien JM, Sibai BM. Daily antenatal testing in women with severe pre-eclampsia. *Am J Obstet Gynecol* 1995;**173**:1207–10.

38. Sezik M, Tuncay G, Yapar EG. Prediction of adverse neonatal outcomes in pre-eclampsia by absent or reversed end-diastolic flow velocity in the umbilical artery. *Gynecol Obstet Invest* 2004;**57**:109–13.

39. Geerts I, Odendaal JH. Severe early onset pre-eclampsia: prognostic value of ultrasound and Doppler assessment. *J Perinatol* 2007;**27**:335–42.

40. Alexander JM, Bloom SL, McIntire DD, Leveno KJ. Severe pre-eclampsia and the very-low birth weight infant: is induction of labor harmful? *Obstet Gynecol* 1999;**93**:485–8.

41. Blackwell SC, Redman ME, Tomlinson M, *et al.* Labor induction for the preterm severe pre-eclamptic patient: is it worth the effort? *J Matern Fetal Med* 2001;**10**:305–11.

42. Hall DR, Odendaal HJ, Steyn DW. Delivery of patients with early onset, severe pre-eclampsia. *Int J Gynecol Obstet* 2001;**74**:143–50.

43. Berkley E, Meng C, Rayburn WF. Success rates with low dose misoprostol before induction of labor for nulliparas with severe pre-eclampsia at various gestational ages. *J Matern Fetal Neonatal Med* 2007;**20**:825–31.

44. Alanis MC, Robinson CJ, Hulsey TC, Ebeling M, Johnson DJ. Early-onset severe pre-eclampsia: induction of labor vs elective cesarean delivery and neonatal outcomes. *Am J Obstet Gynecol* 2008;**199**:262.e1–6.

45. Ascarelli MH, Johnson V, McCreary H, *et al.* Postpartum pre-eclampsia management with furosemide: a randomized clinical trial. *Obstet Gynecol* 2005;**105**:29–33.

Management of eclampsia

10

John T. Repke and Errol R. Norwitz

■ Introduction

Eclampsia refers to the occurrence of one or more generalized grand mal tonic-clonic seizures and/or coma in the setting of preeclampsia and in the absence of underlying neurological disease. The origin of the word is from the Greek "eklampsis," meaning a "shining forth" [1], although other origins have been proposed including "bolt from the blue," a "lightning bolt," and other such terms to describe the aura that commonly precedes the seizure. Eclampsia was at one time thought to be the end result of preeclampsia, hence the nomenclature. It is now clear, however, that seizures are but one clinical manifestation of "severe" preeclampsia.

■ Incidence

Despite recent advances in detection and management, preeclampsia remains the second most common cause of maternal death in the United States (after thromboembolism), accounting for approximately 15% of all maternal deaths [2]. It is estimated that eclampsia is a factor in up to 10% of all maternal deaths in developed countries, and probably accounts for around 50 000 maternal deaths per year worldwide [3].

In the United States and other developed countries, the incidence of eclampsia is relatively stable at around 4–5 per 10 000 live births [4]. In developing countries, however, the reported incidence varies widely from 6–7 to as high as 100 cases per 10 000 live births [5], which reflects in part the lack of adequate prenatal care. Occurrence rates are highest amongst non-white nulliparous women from lower socioeconomic backgrounds.

Hypertension in Pregnancy, ed. Alexander Heazell, Errol R. Norwitz, Louise C. Kenny, and Philip N. Baker. Published by Cambridge University Press. © Cambridge University Press 2010.

Peak incidence is in the teenage years and low twenties, but there is also an increased incidence in women over 35 years of age.

■ Etiology

The pathophysiology of eclampsia is not fully understood, and several possibilities have been proposed (Table 10.1). The two proposed etiologies that have received the most attention are vasospasm and hypertensive encephalopathy. While the definitive etiology remains unproven, these two theories are not mutually exclusive. As preeclampsia worsens, the cerebral circulation is altered. Cerebral autoregulatory mechanisms are designed to maintain cerebral perfusion pressure under circumstances of altered systemic arterial blood pressure. Initially, an increase in systemic blood pressure results in increased cerebral vasoconstriction. However, if the systemic blood pressure exceeds the threshold of the autoregulatory capabilities, then cerebral perfusion pressure and cerebral blood flow increase. This is referred to as segmental arteriolar vasospasm (although it may equally be thought of as segmental arteriolar dilatation) that leads to the development of localized ischemia, increased vascular permeability, cerebral edema, and subsequent seizure activity.

Although eclampsia is a clinical and not a radiological diagnosis, a number of abnormalities are consistently seen on head computed tomography (CT) imaging of eclamptic patients [6] (summarized in Table 10.2). Magnetic resonance (MR) imaging typically shows cerebral changes distributed in a watershed-type pattern, which supports the hypothesis that eclampsia may result from vasospastic-induced global ischemia [7] (Figure 10.1). However, not all eclamptic seizures occur in the setting of markedly elevated systemic blood pressures, suggesting that factors other than disruption of normal cerebral autoregulatory mechanisms are likely

Table 10.1 Possible etiologies of eclamptic convulsions

- Hypertensive encephalopathy
- Cerebrovascular accident
- Cerebral ischemia
- Cerebral infarction
- Cerebral vasospasm
- Cerebral edema
- Microvascular thrombosis
- Metabolic derangement

Table 10.2 Cerebral imaging findings associated with eclampsia

- Cerebral edema
  - Occipital white matter edema
  - Diffuse white matter low density areas
  - Loss of normal cortical sulci
- Cerebral hemorrhage
  - Intraventricular hemorrhage
  - Parenchymal hemorrhage
- Cerebral infarction
  - Basal ganglia infarct
  - Areas of low attenuation

Source: Adapted from: Barton JR, Sibai BM. Cerebral pathology in eclampsia. *Clin Perinatol* 1991;**18**:891–910 [6].

also involved. Results of invasive and functional imaging studies are conflicting. Some angiographic studies have reported widespread vasospasm of the intracranial vessels in patients with eclampsia [8,9], whereas other studies have been unable to confirm this observation [10]. Several investigators have used SPECT (single photon emission CT) and/or positron emission tomography (PET) technology to investigate the neuropathophysiological alterations in eclampsia [10–13], but the data are similarly inconclusive (Figure 10.1).

■ Natural history of eclampsia

Almost half of all cases of eclampsia occur preterm and over one-fifth occur before 31 weeks' gestation [4]. Of those occurring at term, the majority (approximately 75%) occur either intrapartum or within 48 hours of delivery [14]. Traditionally, convulsions occurring more than 48 hours after delivery were not considered eclampsia. However, it is now clear that late postpartum eclampsia (defined as seizures developing greater than 48 hours but before 4 weeks' postpartum) does indeed exist and may account for up to 16% of all cases of eclampsia [15]. Eclampsia prior to 20 weeks' gestation is extremely rare and should raise the possibility of an underlying molar pregnancy, antiphospholipid antibody syndrome, and higher-order multiple pregnancies.

Antepartum cases of eclampsia are often more dramatic than postpartum cases with multiple seizures and maternal complication rates upwards of 70%, including disseminated intravascular coagulopathy

(a)

(b)

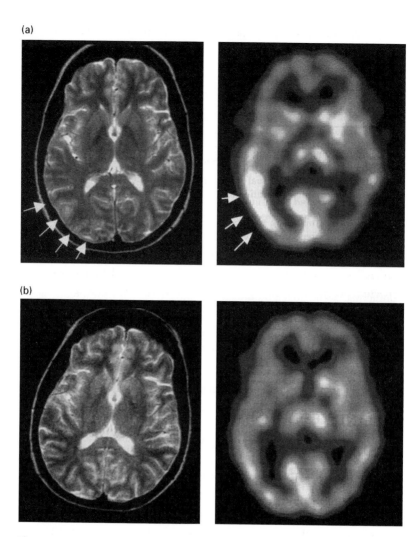

Figure 10.1 Representative head imaging studies of a woman with severe preeclampsia before and after delivery. (a) A representative axial T_2-weighted MRI image (3000 ms/80 ms, TR/TE) of a young woman with severe preeclampsia is shown demonstrating increased T_2 signal (*arrows*) in the peripheral subcortical white matter in the right occipital lobe consistent with hypertensive encephalopathy (left image). A simultaneous axial Tc-99m HMPAO single-photon emission computed tomography image shows increased cerebral perfusion (*arrows*) suggestive of hyperemia in the right posterior temporal cortex, right lateral occipital cortex, and inferior parietal cortex (right image). (b) Follow-up neuroimaging of the same patient eight days after delivery shows marked resolution of both T_2-bright signal on MRI image and of regional hyperperfusion on single-photon emission computed tomography image. See plate section for color version.

(DIC), renal failure, hepatocellular injury, liver rupture, intracerebral hemorrhage, cardiorespiratory arrest, bronchial aspiration, acute pulmonary edema, and postpartum hemorrhage [16].

Prognosis

The reported maternal mortality associated with eclampsia varies from 0.4% to 13.9% [4,16]. In one retrospective analysis of 990 cases, López-Llera reported an overall maternal mortality rate of 13.9% [16]. The highest maternal mortality rate in this cohort (22.2%) was in women with early eclampsia (< 28 weeks). Maternal mortality and severe morbidity rates are lowest among women receiving regular prenatal care who are managed by experienced physicians in tertiary centers [17,18]. The overall perinatal mortality for eclampsia is on the order of 10–25% [4,16]. As expected, perinatal mortality is closely related to gestational age at delivery, and may exceed 90% in pregnant women with eclampsia prior to 28 weeks' gestation [16]. Fetal deaths result primarily from placental abruption, intrauterine asphyxia, and complications of prematurity.

Can we predict an eclamptic seizure?

The relationship between hypertension, symptoms and signs of cortical irritability (headache, visual disturbances, nausea, vomiting, fever, hyperreflexia, clonus), and seizures remains unclear. The majority of women do have one or more antecedent symptoms prior to an eclamptic seizure, including a headache, visual disturbance (scotomata, amaurosis, blurred vision, diplopia, homonymous hemianopsia) or epigastric/upper abdominal pain [4], but the time interval between the symptoms and seizure is often too short to allow for effective seizure prophylaxis. Moreover, in one-third of cases, the seizure is the first manifestation of pregnancy-related hypertensive disease [4].

Although the magnitude of the blood pressure elevation correlates well with the incidence of cerebrovascular accident (stroke), it is not predictive of eclampsia. Indeed, 20–40% of eclamptic patients have no evidence of hypertension prior to their seizure with maximal blood pressures of less than 140/90 mmHg [4,19–21]. In one review by Sibai *et al.* [21] of 179 consecutive cases of eclampsia, the factors found to be at least partially responsible for failure to prevent a seizure were: physician error (36%),

Table 10.3 Differential diagnosis of an eclamptic seizure

- Cerebrovascular accident (e.g., intracerebral hemorrhage, cerebral venous thrombosis)
- Hypertensive diseases (e.g., hypertensive encephalopathy, pheochromocytoma)
- Space-occupying lesions of the central nervous system (e.g., brain tumor, abscess)
- Metabolic disorders (e.g., hypoglycemia, uremia, inappropriate antidiuretic hormone secretion resulting in water intoxication)
- Infectious etiology (e.g., meningitis, encephalitis)
- Thrombotic thrombocytopenic purpura
- Idiopathic epilepsy

magnesium failure (13%), late postpartum onset (12%), early onset (<21 weeks [3%]), abrupt onset (18%), and lack of prenatal care (19%). Therefore, many cases of eclampsia appear not to be preventable, even among women receiving regular prenatal care.

■ Confirming the diagnosis

Eclamptic seizures are clinically and electroencephalographically indistinguishable from other causes of generalized tonic-clonic seizures. Not all women with eclampsia require a head imaging study. However, patients who do not improve following control of seizures and hypertension, those in whom the seizures last longer than 10 minutes, those who have an initial seizure despite being on magnesium sulfate seizure prophylaxis, and those who develop localizing neurological signs should be evaluated further. There is no finding on neuroimaging that is pathognomonic of eclampsia, although the majority of eclamptic women will have transient abnormalities on head CT (most commonly white matter hypodensities in the occipital and parietal regions). The primary goal of the additional testing (including neuroimaging) is therefore to exclude other diagnoses that may mimic eclampsia (Table 10.3).

■ Management of eclampsia

Management of the eclamptic patient can be a challenge given how infrequently it occurs. For this reason, it may be useful for the staff on labor and delivery units with relatively low volumes of high-risk deliveries to periodically participate in exercises on how to approach the acute management of the patient with eclampsia (summarized in Table 10.4).

Table 10.4 Rapid evaluation of the non-hospitalized patient presenting during or after an eclamptic seizure

---

(1) Protect the maternal airway

(2) Protect the mother from injuring herself

(3) Assess fetal condition

(4) Initiate magnesium sulfate seizure prophylaxis

(5) Send off FBC, platelets, AST, ALT, electrolytes, creatinine, blood type and cross match, and urine toxicology screen for illicit drugs

(6) If actively seizing, wait for convulsion to abate and continue with maternal–fetal resuscitation

(7) Formulate a delivery strategy

Note: ALT, alanine transaminase; AST, aspartate transaminase; FBC, full blood count.

Acute management of eclampsia

Not infrequently, the first encounter with the hospital is after a seizure has occurred. These patients often have had scant or no prenatal care, and their presentation to the hospital's emergency department or labor and delivery unit was precipitated by a seizure event at home. In this setting, it is essential that the evaluation of the mother and fetus be swift.

Initial steps at resuscitation should include protecting the mother from injury, protecting her airway, controlling convulsions and blood pressure, prevention of subsequent seizures, assessing the fetal condition and gestational age, and evaluation for delivery. If activity seizing, the woman should be rolled onto her left side and a padded tongue blade placed in her mouth to maintain airway patency and prevent aspiration. The initial laboratory evaluation should include a full blood count (FBC) with platelets, liver, and renal function tests (alanine transaminase [ALT], aspartate transaminase [AST], creatinine), electrolytes, and a urine screen for proteinuria and toxicology, for illicit drugs. The patient should be typed and cross-matched for at least two units of packed red blood cells. Ultrasound should be employed to establish fetal viability and gestational age. If time and circumstances permit, fetal monitoring should be used to better assess the fetal condition.

Eclamptic seizures are almost always self-limiting and seldom last longer than 3 to 4 minutes. As such, it is neither generally necessary nor recommended to intervene to stop the convulsion. However, if the seizure lasts longer than 5 minutes, it is reasonable to administer either magnesium sulfate (2–4 g IV push repeated every 15 minutes to a maximum of 6 g) or a benzodiazepine (such as diazepam 5–10 mg IV push repeated as required to a maximum of 50 mg) to achieve resolution of the ongoing seizure. In the setting of eclampsia, magnesium sulfate is preferred because of the profound respiratory depressant effect of diazepam on the fetus, especially if the total maternal dose exceeds 30 mg. Diazepam-mediated respiratory depression can be intractable and difficult to reverse. As such, immediate access to a clinician skilled in airway management (specifically intubation) is essential if diazepam is used.

If the fetus is alive and of a viable gestational age (> 24 weeks), then strategies for delivery should be developed. At present, an eclamptic seizure is an absolute contraindication to continued expectant management and delivery should be recommended. However, the optimal timing and route of delivery is not known, and recommendations in this regard can be individualized based on generally accepted obstetric indications.

Prevention of recurrent convulsions

Without treatment, approximately 10% of eclamptic women will have repeated seizures [22]. All patients who have experienced an eclamptic seizure require anticonvulsant therapy to prevent recurrent seizures, complications of repeated seizure activity (neuronal death, rhabdomyolysis, metabolic acidosis, aspiration pneumonitis, neurogenic pulmonary edema, and respiratory failure), and possibly cerebrovascular accident. In the United States, the most commonly used medication for the prevention of both primary and recurrent eclamptic seizures is magnesium sulfate. In the absence of specific contraindications to its use, magnesium sulfate should be administered IV using a 4–6 g loading dose over 20 minutes, followed by a continuous IV infusion of 1–2 g per hour [23]. The continuous infusion is given only if a patellar reflex is present (loss of deep tendon reflexes are the first manifestation of symptomatic hypermagnesemia), respirations are greater than 12 per minute, and urine output is greater than 100 mL in four hours. The continuous infusion may also need to be modified based on the patient's renal function, but the loading dose need not be altered. Following serum magnesium levels is not required if the woman's clinical status is closely monitored for evidence of potential magnesium toxicity. If the decision is made to follow serum magnesium levels, the recommended "therapeutic range" is 4.8 to 8.4 mg/dL [24], although it should be remembered that this range has not been tested prospectively. This regimen has been found to be superior to phenytoin [25,26], diazepam [25], nimodipine [27], a "lytic cocktail" (containing promethazine hydrochloride, chlorpromazine, and meperidine hydrochloride) [28], and placebo [29] in preventing eclamptic seizures. Magnesium sulfate therapy also has other advantages. It is cheaper and easier to administer than phenytoin (for which cardiac monitoring is required if given at an infusion rate of $\geq 50\,mg/min$), and it is less sedative than diazepam. Further, magnesium appears to selectively increase cerebral blood flow and oxygen consumption in patients with preeclampsia [30].

Exactly how magnesium acts as an anticonvulsant in eclampsia is not known. Several mechanisms have been proposed, including selective vasodilatation of the cerebral vasculature [30], protection of endothelial cells from damage by free radicals, prevention of calcium ion entry into ischemic cells, and/or as a competitive antagonist to the glutamate N-methyl-D-aspartate receptor (which is epileptogenic).

Anticonvulsant therapy is generally initiated during labor or while administering antenatal corticosteroid therapy or cervical ripening agents prior to a planned delivery in women with severe preeclampsia/eclampsia. Seizure prophylaxis is generally continued for 24 to 48 hours postpartum, at which time the risk of seizures is low.

Management of the hospitalized eclamptic patient

Management of the hospitalized patient who develops eclampsia either prior to or during delivery is somewhat more manageable, but no less frightening. While the majority of hospitalized patients who develop eclampsia will do so intrapartum, some patients may seize while hospitalized for either mild preeclampsia or for severe preeclampsia remote from term that is being managed expectantly. Of late, there has been increasing debate about whether or not magnesium sulfate should be used for seizure prophylaxis in the setting of either mild preeclampsia or preeclampsia that first presents in the postpartum period [23]. The debate goes beyond the scope of this chapter, but it is worth stating that we do not yet have good predictors for who will and who will not go on to develop eclampsia. Most authorities agree that patients with severe preeclampsia or "impending eclampsia" (i.e., women with preeclampsia and symptoms of cortical irritability) should receive intrapartum seizure

Table 10.5 Morbid sequelae of eclampsia

- Maternal apnea
- Fetal asphyxia
- Maternal intracerebral hemorrhage
- Maternal aspiration of gastric contents
- Placental abruption
- Maternal and/or fetal death

Table 10.6 Fetal heart rate changes during an eclamptic seizure

- Fetal bradycardia lasting at least 3 to 5 minutes during the seizure
- Gradual return to baseline as the maternal seizure resolves
- Transient repetitive late decelerations until maternal resuscitation is well under way
- Fetal tachycardia with rate-related reduction in fetal heart rate variability
- Return to a reassuring fetal heart rate tracing within 20 to 30 minutes

prophylaxis with magnesium sulfate [31]. Similarly, since the incidence of seizures is extremely low in women with non-proteinuric pregnancy-induced hypertension (less than 0.1%) [29], it is reasonable to withhold routine seizure prophylaxis in such women.

When a patient experiences an intrapartum eclamptic seizure, the same principles of maternal protection and maternal–fetal resuscitation that were listed above apply. The eclamptic seizure, while dramatic and occasionally terrifying, generally has a predictable course. The best strategy is to wait for the convulsion to abate while maintaining the maternal airway and vital signs. If magnesium sulfate has not yet begun, then it should be started at once. If the patient is already on magnesium sulfate seizure prophylaxis and if there is no evidence of magnesium toxicity, then an additional 2 g IV bolus over 10 minutes should be given. During this time, the mother and fetus should be carefully assessed for the morbid sequelae of eclampsia (Table 10.5).

Fetal heart rate changes are a common finding during and immediately after an eclamptic seizure (Table 10.6). A transient fetal bradycardia lasting at least 3 to 5 minutes can be expected. Resolution of maternal seizure activity is often associated with a compensatory fetal tachycardia and even with transient fetal heart rate decelerations that typically resolve within 20 to 30 minutes [32]. While not entirely preventable, emergent

Table 10.7 Principles of acute management of the intrapartum eclamptic patient

- Avoid emergent Cesarean delivery
- Stabilize mother and fetus
- Initiate or reassess magnesium sulfate seizure prophylaxis
- Assess the cervix, maternal and fetal reserve, and formulate a delivery plan
- Assess and normalize coagulation factors prior to Cesarean delivery, if indicated

Cesarean delivery in the setting of an ongoing eclamptic seizure can place both mother and fetus at increased risk of adverse events, especially if the mother is unstable and general endotracheal anesthesia is used [27]. As such, every attempt should be made to stabilize the mother and resuscitate the fetus in utero before making a decision about delivery.

In the acute setting, it is important also to exclude other potentially catastrophic events such as placental abruption and maternal stroke. In the absence of these relatively rare events, the eclamptic seizure can be managed expectantly and a delivery strategy developed (Table 10.7).

Considerations regarding delivery

Delivery is the only effective treatment for preeclampsia, and eclampsia is an absolute contraindication to continued expectant management. However, immediate delivery does not necessarily imply Cesarean delivery. Indeed, vaginal delivery is generally preferred. A properly managed and successful vaginal delivery is less hemodynamically stressful to the mother and may offer some additional advantages to the term or late preterm infant, such as a lower rate of short-term respiratory complications. It is less clear whether vaginal delivery offers advantages to low and very low birthweight infants. The decision of whether to proceed with Cesarean or induction of labor and attempted vaginal delivery should be individualized based on such factors as parity, gestational age, cervical examination (Bishop score), maternal desire for vaginal delivery, and fetal status and presentation. In general, less than one-third of women with severe preeclampsia remote from term (< 32 weeks' gestation) with an unfavorable cervix will have a successful vaginal delivery [33]. Cervical ripening agents can be used to improve the Bishop score, but prolonged inductions should be avoided.

Adequate pain management is an essential component of any delivery strategy. Regional anesthesia is not contraindicated so long as close attention is paid to volume expansion and anesthetic technique and there is no thrombocytopenia or evidence of coagulopathy. A low platelet count (variably defined as less than 100 000 or less than 75 000 platelets/mm^3 depending on the policy of the individual anesthesiology department) increases the risk of epidural hematoma. Although exceedingly rare, epidural hematomas represent a neurosurgical emergency and may require emergent neurosurgical decompression to prevent permanent spinal nerve injury. With these caveats in mind, epidural analgesia is the preferred mode of pain management in women with preeclampsia/eclampsia. Its slow onset reduces the risk of hypotension (which is a major concern since preeclamptic women are total body fluid overloaded but intravascularly depleted), while the presence of the epidural catheter allows for easy augmentation of analgesia in the event of subsequent Cesarean delivery. General endotracheal anesthesia is best avoided in preeclamptic women because of excessive airway edema and potential exacerbation of hypertension.

Control of blood pressure

Regardless of how or when the patient presents, be it with severe preeclampsia or eclampsia, one critical component of the management is meticulous management of the patient's blood pressure. Aggressive blood pressure control alone in the setting of preeclampsia does not alter the natural course of the disease, does not prevent eclampsia, and does not significantly diminish perinatal morbidity or mortality. For this reason, pharmacological treatment is not generally recommended in preeclamptic women with mild to moderate hypertension. The one clear benefit of aggressive blood pressure control is prevention of cerebrovascular hemorrhage, which is important since stroke accounts for 15–20% of all deaths from eclampsia. The risk of hemorrhagic stroke correlates directly with the degree of elevation in systolic blood pressure and is less related to, but not independent of, the diastolic pressure [34]. It is not clear whether there is a threshold pressure above which emergent therapy should be instituted. Most investigators recommend aggressive antihypertensive therapy for sustained diastolic pressures of ≥ 105–110 mmHg and systolic blood pressures of ≥ 160 mmHg, although these thresholds have not been tested prospectively.

Table 10.8 Pharmacotherapy of acute hypertension in pregnancy

• Hydralazine	5 mg IV push; repeat 5 mg IV push in 10 minutes; then 10 mg IV push every 20 minutes until blood pressure goal achieved. Do not exceed 40 mg (If blood pressure control not achieved by 40 mg change to another agent.)
• Labetalol	5–15 mg IV push; repeat every 10–20 minutes with doubling doses (not exceed 80 mg in any single dose) until a maximum cumulative dose of 300 mg is reached

While systemic arterial pressures may not have a direct effect on the occurrence of eclamptic seizures, the pathophysiology of eclampsia as we currently understand it suggests that careful control of hypertension is important. Several medications may be used to acutely lower blood pressure in this clinical setting, but hydralazine and labetalol are the medications most familiar to obstetricians and, when used intravenously, can generally achieve the appropriate blood pressure goals within a short period of time. In the antepartum or intrapartum patient, it is important not to overcorrect the blood pressure and a goal of 140–150 mmHg systolic and 90–100 mmHg diastolic is deemed to be appropriate. Further reduction in blood pressure may result in relative uteroplacental insufficiency and may not be well tolerated by the fetus. Methods of administration of these two antihypertensive agents are listed in Table 10.8.

■ Atypical eclampsia

Often the diagnosis of eclampsia is readily apparent, but occasionally patients exhibit so-called atypical eclampsia. Examples of atypical eclampsia include cases where there is no diagnosis of preeclampsia, eclampsia prior to 20 weeks of gestation, late postpartum eclampsia (> 4 weeks postpartum), cases in which there are residual focal neurological sequelae, or recurrent refractory seizures despite magnesium sulfate seizure prophylaxis. Depending on the clinical situation, the diagnosis of eclampsia should be entertained until proven otherwise. Magnesium sulfate remains the mainstay of initial anticonvulsant therapy, but it may occasionally be necessary to utilize other agents such as phenytoin or phenobarbital. In such cases, consultation with a neurologist and head imaging studies should be recommended [15].

■ Maternal transport of eclamptic patients

One of the most difficult dilemmas facing the community obstetrician is deciding when to transfer an eclamptic patient to a tertiary care facility. Since eclampsia occurs most often in preterm gestations, the decision to transport the patient is often based on gestational age and the need for a neonatal intensive care unit. It is also important not to forget the maternal condition, which may also be critical. Eclampsia may be accompanied by hypertensive crisis, stroke, and DIC, each of which may require resources available only in a tertiary care facility. Transport should only occur once the patient has been stabilized from a blood pressure and seizure prophylaxis perspective, once fetal viability and well-being has been confirmed, and in a vehicle of sufficient size to allow for appropriate attendance by medical personnel should the patient become unstable en route.

■ Prevention of eclampsia

While many cases of eclampsia can be prevented with timely and appropriate intervention in the setting of preeclampsia, it is clear that prevention is not possible in all cases. Two studies have concluded that eclampsia cannot be prevented in 30–40% of cases even if these patients are hospitalized [17,35]. Fortunately, recurrent eclampsia in a subsequent pregnancy is rare, but is more common in women who develop eclampsia prior to 28 weeks of gestation [36–38].

■ Long-term outcome of women with eclampsia

With the exception of stroke, which often results in long-term neurological sequelae, all other clinical features of preeclampsia/eclampsia resolve following delivery, although this may take several days or even weeks. Diuresis ($>4\,L/day$) is the most accurate clinical indicator of resolution.

Women with a history of preeclampsia have an increased risk of developing a number of conditions in later life, including chronic hypertension [39–41], diabetes mellitus [39,41], end-stage renal disease [42], and cardiovascular disease and death [43]. The risk of developing chronic hypertension remote from preeclampsia ranges from 0% to 78% (average 23.8%) [39–41]. This risk is increased in women who have subsequent hypertensive pregnancies and those with eclampsia remote from term. The wide range in reported risk is due to the influence of variables such as maternal age and duration of follow-up (the increased risk of subsequent hypertension only becomes apparent after an average follow-up of ≥ 10 years [41]). Whether women who develop eclamptic seizures as their manifestation of severe preeclampsia are selectively at risk for these long-term conditions is not known.

■ Conclusion

Eclampsia is a challenge for any clinician in the United States given its relatively low incidence of 4–5 per 10 000 live births. It is an obstetric emergency with both the mother and the fetus at immediate risk for death or life-long neurological disability. Delivery is the only effective treatment. With prompt and effective management and in the absence of cerebrovascular hemorrhage, maternal prognosis is good. Fetal prognosis is dependent largely on gestational age at delivery. Factors that are critical for the successful management of women with eclampsia include:

- Early and regular prenatal care to identify women at risk of eclampsia
- Prompt evaluation and aggressive management of patients presenting with eclampsia, including protecting the patient from injury, maintaining airway protection, adequate ventilation and fluid resuscitation, and rapid assessment of fetal condition
- Meticulous control of blood pressure to avoid stroke
- Seizure prophylaxis with magnesium sulfate
- Stabilizing the maternal condition, resuscitating the fetus in utero, and avoidance of emergent Cesarean delivery, if possible
- Appreciation of other causes of seizures in pregnancy, especially if presenting as "atypical eclampsia"
- Transfer to a tertiary care center when practical
- Appreciation of recurrence risk to facilitate counseling of patients for future pregnancies
- Appreciation of the potential long-term health consequences in women whose pregnancies are complicated by preeclampsia/eclampsia
- Periodic review of eclampsia management with labor and delivery staff.

REFERENCES

1. *Steadman's Medical Dictionary*, 22nd edn. Baltimore, MD, Williams and Wilkins. 1972;392.

2. Rochat RW, Koonin LM, Atrash HF, Jewett JF. Maternal mortality in the United States: Report from the Maternal Mortality Collaborative. *Obstet Gynecol* 1988;**72**:91–7.

3. Duley L. Maternal mortality associated with hypertensive disorders of pregnancy in Africa, Asia, Latin America and the Caribbean. *Br J Obstet Gynaecol* 1992;**99**:547–53.

4. Douglas KA, Redman CWG. Eclampsia in the United Kingdom. *BMJ* 1994;**309**:1395–400.

5. World Health Organization International Collaborative Study of Hypertensive Disorders of Pregnancy. Geographic variation in the incidence of hypertension in pregnancy. *Am J Obstet Gynecol* 1988;**158**:80–3.

6. Barton JR, Sibai BM. Cerebral pathology in eclampsia. *Clin Perinatol* 1991;**18**:891–910.

7. Morriss MC, Twickler DM, Hatab MR, *et al.* Cerebral blood flow and cranial magnetic resonance imaging in eclampsia and severe pre-eclampsia. *Obstet Gynecol* 1997;**89**:561–8.

8. Will AD, Lewis KL, Hinshaw DB, Jr. Cerebral vasoconstriction in toxemia. *Neurology* 1987;**37**:1555–7.

9. Trommer BL, Homer D, Mikhael MA. Cerebral vasospasm and eclampsia. *Stroke* 1988;**19**:326–9.

10. Zunker P, Georgiadis AL, Czech N, *et al.* Impaired cerebral glucose metabolism in eclampsia: a new finding in two cases. *Fetal Diagn Ther* 2003;**18**:41–6.

11. Schwartz RB, Janes KM, Kalina P. Hypertensive encephalopathy: findings on CT, MR imaging, and SPECT imaging in 14 cases. *Am J Roentgenol* 1992;**159**: 379–83.

12. Naidu K, Moodley J, Corr P, Hoffmann M. Single photon emission and cerebral computerised tomographic scan and transcranial Doppler sonographic findings in eclampsia. *Br J Obstet Gynaecol* 1997;**104**:1165–72.

13. Apollon KM, Robinson JN, Schwartz RB, Norwitz ER. Cortical blindness in severe pre-eclampsia: computed tomography, magnetic resonance imaging, and single-photon-emission computed tomography findings. *Obstet Gynecol* 2000;**95**:1017–19.

14. Norwitz ER, Repke JT, Kaplan PW. Eclampsia. In: Gilchrist JM, ed., *Prognosis in Neurology*. Boston, MA, Butterworth-Heinemann. 1998;63–7.

15. Lubarsky SL, Barton JR, Friedman SA, *et al.* Late post-partum eclampsia revisited. *Obstet Gynecol* 1994;**83**:502–5.

16. López-Llera M. Main clinical types and subtypes of eclampsia. *Am J Obstet Gynecol* 1992;**166**:4–9.

17. Sibai BM. Eclampsia. VI. Maternal-perinatal outcome in 254 consecutive cases. *Am J Obstet Gynecol* 1990;**163**:1054–5.

18. Conde-Agudelo A, Kafury-Goeta AC. Case-control study of risk factors for complicated eclampsia. *Obstet Gynecol* 1997;**90**:172–5.

19. Moller B, Lindmark G. Eclampsia in Sweden, 1976–1980. *Acta Obstet Gynecol Scand* 1986;**65**:307–14.

20. Sibai BM, McCubbin JH, Anderson GD, Lipshitz J, Dilts PV, Jr. Eclampsia. I. Observations from sixty-seven recent cases. *Obstet Gynecol* 1981;**58**:609–13.

21. Sibai BM, Abdella TN, Spinnato JA. Eclampsia. V. The incidence of nonpreventable eclampsia. *Am J Obstet Gynecol* 1986;**154**:581–6.

22. Prichard JA, Cunningham FG, Prichard SA. The Parkland Memorial Hospital protocol for treatment of eclampsia: evaluation of 245 cases. *Am J Obstet Gynecol* 1984;**148**:951–63.

23. American College of Obstetricians and Gynecologists. *Diagnosis and Management of Pre-eclampsia and Eclampsia.* ACOG Practice Bulletin No. 33. Washington, DC, ACOG, 2002.

24. Sibai BM, Lipshitz J, Anderson GD, Dilts PV, Jr. Reassessment of intravenous MgSO4 therapy in preeclampsia-eclampsia. *Obstet Gynecol* 1981;**57**:199–202.

25. The Eclampsia Trial Collaborative Group. Which anticonvulsant for women with eclampsia? Evidence from the Collaborative Eclampsia Trial. *Lancet* 1995;**345**:1455–63.

26. Lucas MJ, Leveno KJ, Cunningham FG. A comparison of magnesium sulfate with phenytoin for the prevention of eclampsia. *N Engl J Med* 1995;**333**:201–5.

27. Belfort MA, Anthony J, Saade GR, Allen JC, Jr. for the Nimodipine Study Group. A comparison of magnesium sulfate and nimodipine for the prevention of eclampsia. *N Engl J Med* 2003;**348**:304–11.

28. Duley L, Gulmezoglu AM. Magnesium sulfate versus lytic cocktail for eclampsia. *Cochrane Database Syst Rev* 2001;(1):CD002960.

29. Coetzee EJ, Dommisse J, Anthony J. A randomised controlled trial of intravenous magnesium sulphate versus placebo in the management of women with severe pre-eclampsia. *Br J Obstet Gynaecol* 1998;**105**:300–3.

30. Belfort MA, Moise KJ, Jr. Effect of magnesium sulfate on maternal brain blood flow in pre-eclampsia: a randomized, placebo-controlled study. *Am J Obstet Gynecol* 1992;**167**:661–6.

31. Repke JT. Pre-eclampsia and hypertension. In: Repke JT, ed., *Intrapartum Obstetrics.* New York, NY, Churchill Livingstone. 1996;253–73.

32. Paul RH, Koh KS, Bernstein SG. Changes in fetal heart rate-uterine contraction patterns associated with eclampsia. *Am J Obstet Gynecol* 1978;**130**:165–9.

33. Nassar AH, Adra AM, Chakhtoura N. Severe pre-eclampsia remote from term: labor induction or elective cesarean delivery? *Am J Obstet Gynecol* 1998;**179**:1210–13.

34. Lindenstrom E, Boysen G, Nyboe J. Influence of systolic and diastolic blood pressure on stroke risk: a prospective observational study. *Am J Epidemiol* 1995;**142**:1279–90.

35. Campbell DM, Templeton AA. Is eclampsia preventable? In: Bonner J, MacGillivray I, Symonds EM, eds., *Pregnancy Hypertension.* Baltimore, MD, University Park Press. 1980;483–8.

36. Chesley LC, Cosgrove RA, Annitto JE. A follow-up study of eclamptic women. *Am J Obstet Gynecol* 1962;**83**:1360–72.

37. Lopez-Llera M, Hernández Horta JL. Pregnancy after eclampsia. *Am J Obstet Gynecol* 1974;**119**:193–8.

38. Adelusi B, Ojengbede OA. Reproductive performance after eclampsia. *Int J Gynaecol Obstet* 1986;**24**:183–9.

39. Chesley LC, Annitto JE, Cosgrove RA. The remote prognosis of eclamptic women. *Am J Obstet Gynecol* 1976;**124**:446–59.

40. Sibai BM, Sarinoglu C, Mercer BM. Eclampsia. VII. Pregnancy after eclampsia and long-term prognosis. *Am J Obstet Gynecol* 1992;**166**:1757–61.

41. Sibai BM, el-Nazer A, Gonzalez-Ruiz A. Severe pre-eclampsia-eclampsia in young primigravid women: subsequent pregnancy outcome and remote prognosis. *Am J Obstet Gynecol* 1986;**155**:1011–16.

42. Vikse BE, Irgens LM, Leivestad T, Skjaerven R, Iversen BM. Pre-eclampsia and the risk of end-stage renal disease. *N Engl J Med* 2008;**359**:800–9.

43. Funai EF, Friedlander Y, Paltiel O, *et al*. Long-term mortality after pre-eclampsia. *Epidemiology* 2005;**16**:206–15.

Anesthesia in preeclampsia

11

John Clift and Alexander Heazell

■ Introduction

Anesthetists should be informed of all patients with preeclampsia admitted to the labor ward and review these patients at the earliest opportunity. Anesthetic input is involved for the following aspects of care:

- To provide analgesia for labor
- To assess the patient before any operative procedure
- To provide anesthesia for operative procedures including Cesarean section, the incidence of which is increased in preeclampsia
- To assess the need for and provide invasive monitoring
- To manage eclamptic fits as part of a multidisciplinary team
- To provide medical management of preeclampsia/eclampsia as part of the multidisciplinary team.

■ Epidural analgesia for labor

This is considered the best mode of analgesia for patients with preeclampsia for the following reasons:

- It lowers the blood pressure and attenuates the hypertensive response to pain
- It provides excellent analgesia
- It can be used for operative delivery
- Increases intervillous (placental) blood flow provided hypotension is avoided
- Reduces the maternal stress response.

It is best to use a low-dose mixture of local anesthetic + opiates (e.g., 0.1% bupivacaine + 2 mcg/mL fentanyl), as this produces less hypotension and

Hypertension in Pregnancy, ed. Alexander Heazell, Errol R. Norwitz, Louise C. Kenny, and Philip N. Baker. Published by Cambridge University Press. © Cambridge University Press 2010.

preserves motor function reducing the incidence of instrumental vaginal delivery. The mixture may be administered by midwife top-ups, PCEA (patient controlled epidural analgesia) or continuous infusion of the epidural solution.

Intravenous access should be established with a large-bore cannula. In severe preeclampsia, intravenous fluids should be minimized to reduce the risk of pulmonary edema. In the event of hypotension, which is rare in the low-dose epidural regime, the management should consist of the following:

- Turn the patient into the left lateral position
- High flow oxygen
- Small bolus of fluids, e.g., 250 mL crystalloid
- Intravenous vasopressor boluses, e.g., ephedrine 3 mg or phenylephrine 50 mcg. Care should be taken, due to the increased response to vasopressors in preeclamptic patients.

Rather than the absolute drop in blood pressure, the hypotensive effect on the cardiotocograph (CTG), which should be monitored continuously, may be more significant.

■ Preoperative assessment

An accurate clinical assessment of patients with preeclampsia is essential, as dysfunction of most organ systems will impact on anesthetic management. Of particular importance to the anesthetist are the following.

Respiratory system

The presence of facial edema, a hoarse voice, shortness of breath, and stridor should alert the anesthetist to the possibility of laryngeal edema and difficult intubation.

Hypoxia, shortness of breath, and fine inspiratory crackles at the lung bases indicate pulmonary edema.

Cardiovascular system

The blood pressure should be assessed and controlled prior to anesthesia, because of the potential risks to the mother of an intracerebral hemorrhage. Such events were responsible for the majority of maternal deaths in patients with preeclampsia in the UK between 2005 and 2007 [1].

Following analysis of these cases the Confidential Enquiry into Maternal and Child Health (CEMACH) suggests the systolic blood pressure is reduced to < 160 mmHg and it would seem sensible to keep the diastolic blood pressure < 100mmHg, to reduce the incidence of maternal hypertensive crises [2]. Consideration should be given to commencing treatment at lower blood pressures if other evidence of severe preeclampsia is present and severe hypertension may be anticipated. The importance of blood pressure control takes precedence over fetal well-being [2]. This principle is of particular importance when a general anesthetic is planned.

Central nervous system

Most patients with severe preeclampsia are treated with intravenous magnesium sulfate. This is of particular significance for patients having a general anesthetic as it may reduce the fasciculations observed with suxamethonium and prolong the action of non-depolarizing muscle relaxants, thus necessitating the use of a nerve stimulator to assess muscle relaxation.

A nerve stimulator is a monitoring device that measures the degree of muscle relaxation (paralysis) by transcutaneously stimulating a peripheral nerve. Most commonly used is the ulnar nerve, at the wrist, and the response is detected by observing thumb adduction.

Coagulation cascade

The patient with preeclampsia may have an abnormal platelet count, platelet function, or prolonged clotting. This may increase the risk of epidural hematoma when a regional anesthetic technique is used. Patients with preeclampsia should have had a platelet count within the 12 hours prior to having regional anesthesia/analgesia (6 hours if rapid deterioration). Whilst there is no consensus as what constitutes a safe level of platelets for regional techniques, the following would seem a reasonable approach; a platelet count of:

- $> 100\,000 \times 10^9$/L, it is safe to proceed with a regional technique
- $80\,000–100\,000 \times 10^9$/L, clotting studies should also be done. It is safe to proceed if the international normalized ratio (INR) and activated partial thromboplastin time (APTTR) are < 1.5
- $< 80\,000 \times 10^9$/L is considered a relative contraindication to a regional technique (see paragraph below).

The above should be used as a guide only and the risk of performing regional anesthesia/analgesia with abnormal clotting should be weighed up against the benefit, particularly the avoidance of general anesthesia. The risk of developing an epidural hematoma is very small, but its potential consequences (paralysis) can be devastating.

■ Anesthesia for Cesarean section

Spinal

In preeclamptic patients without a working epidural; spinal or combined spinal-epidural (CSE) anesthesia is the anesthetic of choice for Cesarean section, because it avoids general anesthesia and its associated risks. Initial concerns that hypotension may be worse in preeclamptic patients receiving spinal anesthesia, as opposed to healthy parturients, have proved unfounded and these patients may in fact have less hypotension [3]. The severity of hypotension after spinal and epidural anesthesia appears to be similar [4].

The anesthetic used should consist of a local anesthetic and opiate, this should be no different to that used in a healthy patient having a Cesarean section and should provide a sensory block to T4 (cold) and T5 (touch).

The principle of fluid balance is to restrict fluid input during the operation. Preloading is best avoided as there are minimal benefits and extra fluid increases the risk of developing pulmonary edema. Intraoperative hypotension is best treated with intravenous vasopressor boluses, e.g., phenylephrine 50 mcg or ephedrine 3 mg; care should be taken when giving these drugs as some patients have an exaggerated hypertensive response to them. Blood loss during Cesarean section should be promptly replaced with intravenous fluids initially and blood, if the loss is large enough. Fluid balance in these patients can be particularly difficult and if blood loss is severe or ongoing, invasive monitoring should be instituted earlier than in non-preeclamptic patients.

Epidural

A working epidural for labor can be topped up to provide anesthesia, and is the anesthetic of choice in preeclamptic patients. Incremental doses of a mixture of bupivacaine 0.5% ± fentanyl are suitable. The required block height, fluid management, and treatment of hypotension are as for spinal anesthesia (described previously). The advantage of epidural anesthesia (and CSE) is that it can be used to provide postoperative analgesia. This may minimize lability of blood pressure postoperatively.

General anesthesia

General anesthesia is best avoided in the preeclamptic patient because of the increased risks, however, it may be required in cases where regional anesthesia has failed or is contraindicated, e.g., coagulopathy.

The risk of difficult intubation is increased in the preeclamptic patient because of the risk of laryngeal edema. Therefore the airway should be assessed and the anesthetist must be prepared, as in all obstetric cases, for a difficult intubation. In cases where there is obvious laryngeal edema, alternative methods of securing an airway should be used, e.g., awake direct or fiber-optic intubation. The reason for not using regional anesthesia should also be revisited. Nasal intubation is best avoided because of the risk of bleeding. It must also be remembered that laryngeal edema may develop during the anesthetic (trauma of intubation or progression of disease) and therefore prior to extubation the endotracheal cuff should be let down to make sure there is a cuff leak. In the event of a failed intubation, siting and securing a surgical airway may be more difficult due to the presence of facial edema.

There is an exaggerated pressor response to intubation in the preeclamptic patient increasing the risk of cerebrovascular accident (the largest cause of mortality in the preeclamptic patient), cardiac arrhythmias, pulmonary edema, and reduced uterine blood flow. The anesthetist should anticipate an additional rise in blood pressure at intubation and be given as much time as possible to try and prevent the pressor effects of intubation even when there are pressing fetal reasons for urgent Cesarean section under general anesthesia [2]. Methods used for obtunding this response include: intravenous alfentanil (10 mcg/kg), lignocaine (1.5 mg/kg), magnesium (40 mg/kg), or labetalol (10–20 mg) [4], prior to induction. Care should be taken to obtund the response to extubation, which may also be exaggerated; esmolol or labetalol may be used for this purpose. Careful consideration should be given to the use of invasive arterial blood pressure monitoring.

The implications of magnesium sulfate treatment for neuromuscular blockade in general anesthesia have already been mentioned.

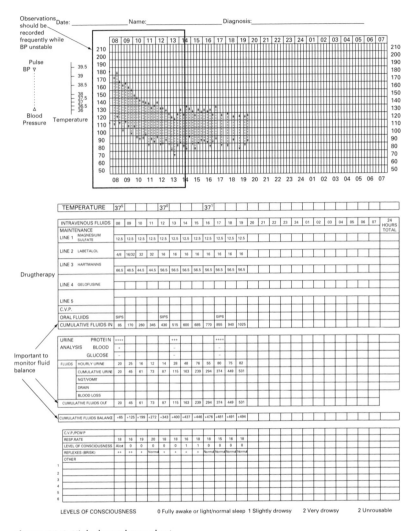

Figure 11.1 High-dependency chart.

■ Monitoring

Patients with severe preeclampsia or eclampsia require regular monitoring of blood pressure, urine output, and oxygen saturation and should be managed in a 1:1 setting, i.e., a level 1 or 2 care area. The use of a high-dependency chart provides a valuable overview of the patient's condition, and should contain information on blood pressure, pulse, respiratory rate, temperature, fluids in, fluid output, and reflexes (Figure 11.1).

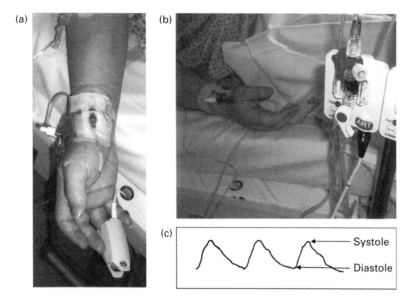

Figure 11.2 Invasive blood pressure monitoring via radial arterial cannula. (a) Arterial cannula in right radial artery. (b) Transducer for recording of the arterial pulse wave. (c) Example of arterial pulse wave obtained in radial artery. Images reproduced with patients' permission.

Invasive blood pressure monitoring

Cannulation of the radial artery (most commonly used site) is usually performed to allow direct monitoring of the blood pressure (Figure 11.2). The advantages are that it allows continuous assessment of the blood pressure and arterial blood sampling.

It is indicated in patients who have an unstable blood pressure. In preeclamptic patients this includes:

• Those whose blood pressure has been labile due to antihypertensive treatment.

• Those on large doses of antihypertensive treatment, particularly on addition of a second intravenous antihypertensive agent. The combination may cause large swings in blood pressure.

• Those on antihypertensive treatment who have had a significant blood loss. The need for an arterial line would occur at a lower blood loss compared to the non-preeclamptic patient.

It is also indicated in preeclamptic patients requiring regular blood gas analysis, e.g., hypoxia.

One must balance the above-mentioned benefits against the complications associated with its use, these include: hematoma, distal ischemia, infection, pseudoaneurysm, accidental injection of drugs, and bleeding from accidental disconnection. Arterial lines should only be looked after by appropriately trained personnel, and this usually means the patient should be cared for in a level 2 or level 3 critical care facility.

■ Fluid management

Fluid balance must be carefully monitored in women with severe preeclampsia due to the possibility of pulmonary and renal sequelae. It should be noted that the incidence of pulmonary complications is greater than renal dysfunction or failure.

Renal

Preeclampsia is often associated with a reduction in glomerular filtration rate and effective renal plasma flow. In most cases this reverses within 48 hours of delivery. Prerenal acute renal failure (ARF) occurs because of decreased renal perfusion. Prompt correction of this will reverse the condition and prevent progression to intrarenal ARF and possible long-term kidney damage. The goal of intravenous fluid therapy is to reverse pre-ischemic changes and prevent further damage. As renal perfusion decreases, a functioning kidney acts by conserving sodium, thus decreasing renal excretion of sodium in the urine.

Respiratory

The reasons preeclamptic patients are at risk of pulmonary edema are best described by Starling's forces which determine the amount of fluid moving across an endothelium

$$Q = K\,[(P_c - P_i) - \sigma(\pi_c - \pi_i)]$$

Q is flow across the endothelium for a given surface area
K is the flow per unit pressure gradient across the endothelium (filtration coefficient)
P_c is capillary hydrostatic pressure
P_i is interstitial fluid hydrostatic pressure

σ is the reflection coefficient which represents capillary "leakiness" to plasma proteins

π_c is the plasma oncotic pressure

π_i is the interstitial fluid oncotic pressure.

It has been demonstrated in preeclamptic patients that the following occur:

- The pulmonary capillary wedge pressure (PCWP) is increased. This corresponds to P_c and is elevated due to mobilization of fluid from the extravascular to intravascular space after delivery and the administration of fluid.
- π_c is reduced due to the reduced level of plasma proteins most notably albumin. Hypoalbuminemia (< 25 mg/L) is common in severe preeclampsia.
- σ is reduced due to endothelial cell damage, i.e., there is increased "leakiness."

It can therefore be seen that the above three factors all act to increase Q, i.e., the flow of fluid across the endothelium and therefore increase the risk of developing pulmonary edema.

Management of fluid balance

The aim of fluid management is to fluid restrict patients, to reduce the risk of pulmonary edema, because the risk of developing pulmonary edema is relatively common compared with ARF or other end-organ damage. Pulmonary edema is associated with significant morbidity and mortality. Commonly, women are restricted to 80–85 mL/h of fluid, which has been associated with good outcome [5]; this is the volume for total fluid intake and includes intravenous, oral, and infusions.

Triggers for intervention

Ideally there would be a physiological parameter which could be measured, and acts as a trigger for fluid administration. In the past the urine output has been used to monitor response but there is no good evidence that aiming for a specific urine output is important to prevent renal failure [2]. Other markers that could be used include plasma creatinine or urinary sodium; further work needs to be done to show whether these are appropriate and at what level the trigger point should be.

Clinical examination

Patients with any evidence of pulmonary edema should not have further fluid boluses. Therefore, the chest should be auscultated prior to each fluid bolus, and signs of pulmonary edema preclude the use of fluid. In the presence of preeclampsia a low oxygen saturation (SaO_2) raises a high index of suspicion that pulmonary edema has developed. Oxygen should be given and intravenous frusemide considered for the treatment of pulmonary edema.

Monitoring intervention response

The ideal method of monitoring the response to fluid administration should be able to inform us if the patient is fluid responsive, i.e., the stroke volume increases in response to a fluid bolus. Several other monitoring strategies have been used including hourly urine output, invasive monitoring of central venous pressure (CVP), or PCWP.

Hourly urine output

Strict fluid balance charts, showing fluid input and output, should be kept on all patients with severe preeclampsia. To facilitate the measurement of urine output the patient will require an indwelling urinary catheter. However, there is insufficient evidence that aiming for a specific urine output will prevent renal damage or failure [2]. Current guidelines propose that oliguria is defined as < 0.5 mL/kg/h for 4 hours.

CVP

Central venous pressure is most commonly measured via a catheter situated in the internal jugular vein, the subclavian vein may also be used. The CVP is commonly used to direct fluid therapy. Absolute CVP measurements fail to estimate the response to fluid in at least 50% of patients. A low CVP does not mean that the patient will respond to fluids. The CVP has also been used to dynamically assess the response to fluid boluses, i.e., fluid is administered and changes in of the CVP assessed. However, there is a very weak relationship between CVP and fluid volume. Hence, an isolated CVP reading does not indicate a low intravascular volume. In addition, there is a weak relationship between CVP (both single readings and changes in CVP) and the hemodynamic response to a fluid challenge. In preeclampsia there is a poor correlation between CVP readings and left-heart filling pressures [6]. Therefore, CVP monitoring cannot measure fluid response as defined by an increase in stroke volume following a fluid bolus. As such, CVP should not be used to make clinical decisions regarding fluid management in patients with preeclampsia [7]. Complications of central venous line insertion include: pneumothorax, arterial puncture, air embolism, arrhythmias, sepsis, and thrombosis.

Pulmonary arterial catheterization

The pulmonary artery catheter has been used in managing patients with severe preeclampsia. However, there are several problems associated with its use.

It is an invasive method of monitoring; a sheath is introduced into the subclavian or internal jugular vein. The catheter is introduced through this, connected to a pressure transducer, and the balloon at its tip inflated. This tip advanced into the right atrium, through the right ventricle, and into the pulmonary artery, guided by the pressure waveform changes detected by the transducer. The PCWP is revealed by a characteristic waveform and the balloon is deflated. The PCWP reflects left atrial pressure. Complications include: the complications of CVP insertion (see above) and arrhythmias including heart block, knotting of the catheter, pulmonary infarction, and pulmonary artery rupture. There is a greater incidence of complications as compared with CVP insertion. Its use has declined as has the experience of clinicians. Fluid management should be guided by fluid responsiveness, i.e., stroke volume response to fluid, rather than one-off pressure (PCWP) readings. It should therefore be used as a cardiac output monitor. The main problem with its use is that it has never been shown to improve survival in the critically ill patient [8], or improve the outcome of the mother or fetus [9]. Its routine use cannot be recommended.

Cardiac output monitors

There are several different types of cardiac output monitors. Many of these are less invasive and have been validated by comparing them to the pulmonary artery catheter. These usually measure stroke volume indirectly and can therefore be used to determine whether a patient is fluid responsive or not. An in-depth discussion regarding their use is beyond the scope of this chapter but they may become increasingly used in the future.

Intervention for low urine output

In the patient who has impending ARF, treatment is required to avoid the need for hemodialysis/hemofiltration and potential long-term damage. The aim is to increase cardiac output by intravenous fluid administration and thus improve blood flow to the kidneys. All patients given a fluid bolus are at increased risk of developing pulmonary edema but only those who are "fluid responders" have the potential to benefit from such a treatment. A fluid bolus should be given to patients who are fluid responders and a period of time, e.g., 4–6 hours, should be allowed to elapse before assessing the response to that fluid. An inadequate response may necessitate further fluid administration.

Furosemide should not be given to treat oliguria because it is not associated with any significant clinical benefits in the prevention and treatment of ARF. High doses may be associated with an increase risk of ototoxicity [10]. It may also worsen the situation where the oliguria is caused by hypovolemia or dehydration.

Dopamine increases urine output but should not be used as it showed no differences in plasma creatinine [11], need for renal replacement therapy (RRT), or length of hospital/intensive care unit stay [12].

Plasma expansion

There is no evidence to support the routine use of maternal volume expansion, the process of improving maternal organ perfusion by expanding the plasma volume. It does not improve outcome in preeclampsia, but it may induce pulmonary edema [13].

■ Admission to the critical care unit

The patient who develops significant pulmonary edema should be transferred to a critical care unit for further respiratory support; this will include closer monitoring, intravenous furosemide, continuous positive airway pressure (CPAP), or intermittent positive pressure ventilation (IPPV).

The indications for RRT would include: pulmonary edema not responsive to diuretics, an elevated rising potassium, worsening metabolic acidosis, and symptomatic uremia. Admission to a critical care unit would normally have occurred before the patient reaches this stage.

■ Managing eclampsia

Eclampsia describes fits, convulsions, or coma without the presence of an underlying reason after 20 weeks of pregnancy (covered in more depth in Chapter 10). Eclamptic fits are usually generalized tonic-clonic seizures lasting 1–2 minutes. They are usually self-limiting. Importantly, eclampsia may occur prior to the onset of symptoms and signs of preeclampsia.

The acute management of eclamptic fit requires anesthetic input, particularly to maintain a patent airway. The basic principles are
- **A**irway
- **B**reathing
- **C**irculation
- IV access should be obtained
- 4 g magnesium sulfate is used to control the seizure followed by a maintenance infusion as described for severe preeclampsia (see Chapter 9)
- For recurrent seizures a further 2 g bolus of magnesium is given and the maintenance increased to 20 mL/h (2 g/h)
- Rarely, seizures may be resistant to magnesium sulfate. The use of intravenous diazepam is then warranted, if this fails thiopentone may be required. The latter requires intubation and admission to the critical care unit.

■ Managing severe preeclampsia/eclampsia as part of a multidisciplinary team

Less than 8% of patients with severe preeclampsia/HELLP (hemolysis, elevated liver enzymes, and low platelets) syndrome and 10% of patients with eclampsia develop significant or multiple organ dysfunction necessitating invasive monitoring and treatment [14,15]. It is essential that anesthetic staff are involved in patient care as early as possible in order that patients are cared for in the most appropriate clinical area, which may be in another unit. Therefore, all health professionals should understand the different levels of care to facilitate effective communication between professionals involved in patient care.

Definitions

Level 0: Patients whose needs can be met through normal ward care

Level 1: Patients at risk of deteriorating, whose needs can be met on an acute ward with the help of outreach/critical care team

Level 2: Patients requiring more detailed observations or interventions including support for a single failing organ. This is also known as a high dependency unit (HDU)

Level 3: Patients requiring advanced respiratory support alone, or the support of at least two organ systems. This is also known as an intensive or critical care unit.

In the UK, many maternity units have areas of higher care, often reflecting a better midwifery to patient ratio or midwives with advanced training. It is important to establish whether these are level 1 or 2. The term "high dependency unit" has been used to cover both these areas and is not a clinically useful term. Level of care is better defined by 0–3 rather than the terms HDU and ICU. The decision regarding the level of care required should be made on an individual basis by an experienced obstetrician, anesthetist, and intensivist with input from specialist physicians when required.

Admission criteria for level 1 care

Patients:

- Discharged from more advanced levels of support
- Requiring additional monitoring, e.g., observations more frequently than 4 hourly, pulse oximetry, fluid input/output
- Requiring additional clinical input, e.g., reflexes, magnesium sulfate, coagulopathy
- In whom there are concerns regarding their physical condition.

If there is any doubt, place the patient in the higher level of care.

Admission criteria for level 2 care

Patients:

- Requiring monitoring that cannot be safely provided in level 1 care
- Requiring respiratory support, e.g., $> 40\%$ O_2, non-invasive ventilation, CPAP, respiratory rate > 25/min
- With hemodynamic instability, intra-arterial BP monitoring, or having antihypertensive drug infusions

- With Glasgow Coma Score < 14
- Requiring haemofiltration.

Admission criteria for level 3 care

Patients requiring:

- Advanced respiratory monitoring or support, e.g., IPPV
- Monitoring or support of two or more organs, e.g., intravenous medication to control seizures and supplementary oxygen/airway monitoring.

REFERENCES

1. Lewis GE. (ed.) The Confidential Enquiry into Maternal and Child Health, *Saving Mothers' Lives: reviewing maternal deaths to make motherhood safer – 2003–2005*. The Seventh Report of the Confidential Enquiries into Maternal Deaths in the United Kingdom. London, CEMACH, 2007.
2. Royal College of Obstetricians and Gynaecologists. *The Management of Severe Pre-eclampsia/Eclampsia. Green Top Guideline 10A*. London, RCOG Press, 2006.
3. Aya AG, Mangin R, Vialles N, *et al*. Patients with severe preeclampsia experience less hypotension during spinal anesthesia for elective caesarean delivery than healthy parturients: a prospective cohort comparison. *Anesth Analg* 2003;**97**: 867–872.
4. Hart C, Coley S. The diagnosis and management of pre-eclampsia. Continuing education in anesthesia, *Crit Care Pain* 2003;**3**:38–42.
5. Tuffnell DJ, Jankowicz D, Lindlow SW, *et al*. Outcomes of severe preeclampsia/ eclampsia in Yorkshire 1999–2003. *Br J Obstet Gynaecol* 2005;**112**:875–80.
6. Bolte AC, Dekker GA, van Eyck J, van Schijndel RS, van Geijn HP. Lack of agreement between central venous pressure and pulmonary capillary wedge pressure in pre-eclampsia. *Hypertens Pregnancy* 2000;**19**:261–71.
7. Marik PE, Baram M, Vahid B. Does central venous pressure predict fluid responsiveness?: a systematic review of the literature and the tale of seven mares. *Chest* 2008;**134**:172–8.
8. Wheeler AP, Bernard GR, Thompson BT, *et al*. Pulmonary-artery versus central venous catheter to guide treatment of acute lung injury. *N Engl J Med* 2006;**354**:2213–24.
9. Brodie H, Malinow AM. Anesthetic management of preeclampsia/eclampsia. *Int J Obstet Anesth* 1998;**8**:110–24.
10. Ho KM, Sheridan DJ. Meta-analysis of frusemide to prevent or treat acute renal failure. *BMJ* 2006;**333**:420–5.
11. Steyn DW, Steyn P. Low dose dopamine for women with severe preeclampsia. *Cochrane Database Syst Rev* 2007;(1):CD003515.

12. ANZICS Clinical Trials Group. Low dose dopamine in patients with early renal dysfunction: a placebo controlled randomised trial. *Lancet* 2000;356: 2139–43.

13. Duley L, Williams J, Henderson-Smart DJ. Plasma volume expansion for treatment of pre-eclampsia. *Cochrane Database Syst Rev* 2000;(2):CD001805 DOI:10.1002/14651858. CD001805.

14. Sibai B, Ramadan MK, Usta I, *et al.* Maternal morbidity and mortality in 442 pregnancies with hemolysis, elevated liver enzymes, and low platelets (HELLP syndrome). *Am J Obstet Gynecol* 1993;**169**(4):1000–6.

15. Bhagwanjee S, Paruk F, Moodley J, Muckhart DJ. Intensive care unit morbidity and mortality from eclampsia: an evaluation of the Acute Physiology and Chronic Health Evaluation II score and the Glasgow Coma Scale score. *Crit Care Med* 2000;**28**(1):120–4.

FURTHER READING

Levy DM. Anaesthesia for Caesarean Section. *Cont Educ Anaesth Crit Care Pain* 2001;**1**:171–6.

Long-term significance following hypertension in pregnancy

12

Stephen Thung and Edmund F. Funai

■ Introduction

Obstetricians have long known that women with pregnancies complicated by medical diseases such as diabetes, renal insufficiency, and hypertension are at increased risk for common obstetrical complications such as preeclampsia, preterm birth, and fetal growth abnormalities. With the exception of gestational diabetes, conventional wisdom long held that pregnancy complications were self-limited and the implications of obstetrical complications on future maternal life have been largely overlooked. As such, research has traditionally focused upon the link between adult-onset chronic diseases of the offspring during pregnancies complicated by fetal disorders like intrauterine growth restriction and macrosomia (the "fetal programing" hypothesis) [1]. A growing body of research now suggests a new concern; that obstetrical conditions such as preeclampsia should be viewed as risk factors for later cardiovascular disease (CVD) and should be used in a similar fashion as family history and body mass index. Perhaps events during pregnancy may be used as a "crystal ball" to peer into the future and identification of pregnancy complications by primary care physicians may be a unique screening opportunity for future care [2].

Hypertension in Pregnancy, ed. Alexander Heazell, Errol R. Norwitz, Louise C. Kenny, and Philip N. Baker. Published by Cambridge University Press. © Cambridge University Press 2010.

■ Preeclampsia and later-life cardiovascular disease: observational data

Until recently, most authorities believed that preeclampsia was not associated with significant long-term health problems. However, the National High Blood Pressure Education Program's Working Group on High Blood Pressure during Pregnancy has asserted that unusual circumstances, such as recurrent hypertension in pregnancy, preeclampsia in a multiparous woman, or early-onset disease in any pregnancy, may be associated with future health risks [3].

Current knowledge of any potential long-term sequelae may have been first appreciated in 1976 by Dr. Leon Chesley, who initially detailed the outcomes of women with eclampsia in their first pregnancy. He found no increased hypertension risk or death in these women. However, he did demonstrate a two- to fivefold excess mortality over the next 35 years among women with eclampsia in any pregnancy beyond the first [4]. He suspected astutely that future mortality was not determined by having preeclampsia/eclampsia but due to underlying chronic hypertension, and that this underlying disease was responsible for the subsequent increase in morbidity and mortality. These suspicions were confirmed by Sibai *et al.* who later demonstrated that apparently healthy women with recurrent preeclampsia were more likely to develop overt chronic hypertension. This relationship was further strengthened if a woman had preterm preeclampsia during pregnancy [5].

Large cohort experiences have reinforced Chesley's conclusions. A Norwegian cohort involving over 626 000 births demonstrated a modestly increased risk for cardiovascular mortality (risk ratio [RR], 1.65; 95% confidence interval [CI], 1.01–2.70) in women with term preeclampsia and an even stronger association (RR, 8.12; 95% CI, 4.31–15.33) with preterm preeclampsia requiring early delivery [6]. Scottish investigators confirmed this finding with their own 129 000 patient cohort and found a modest increase in death related to ischemic heart disease (RR, 1.7; 95% CI, 0.9–3.3). Again, a synergistic effect was noted when preeclampsia occurred preterm (RR, 6.4; 95% CI, 1.9–21.3) and further increased when the lowest birthweight quintile was factored (RR, 16.1; 95% CI, 3.6–72.6) [7]. Funai and colleagues described excess long-term mortality in a cohort of Israeli women with prior preeclampsia. Compared with women who were not diagnosed with preeclampsia, the relative risk of death after preeclampsia was 2.1 (95% CI, 1.8–2.5). Deaths from CVD contributed most strongly to this increase, a threefold increase. Interestingly, among women with preeclampsia who had subsequent births without preeclampsia, the excess risk of mortality became manifest only after 20 years [8].

Preeclampsia may also be associated with the development of end-stage renal disease (ESRD). A Norwegian experience of 570 433 women demonstrated that first pregnancy preeclampsia was associated with ESRD (RR, 4.7; 95% CI, 3.6–6.1). A dose-dependent relationship was seen with the risk for ESRD in two pregnancies with preeclampsia being 6.4-fold increased (95% CI, 3.0–13.5). With two or three pregnancies complicated by preeclampsia the risk was highest (RR, 15.5; 95% CI, 7.8–30.8) [9]. Fortunately, the absolute risk remains low.

Most recently, Lykke *et al.* [10] studied the association between hypertensive disorders of pregnancy and adverse health outcomes in a national Danish cohort of women who delivered between 1978 and 2007 with singleton pregnancies (n = 782 287) and two consecutive singleton deliveries (n = 536 419). They demonstrated increasing risks with severity of disease from: (1) gestational (pregnancy-induced) hypertension, (2) mild preeclampsia, and (3) severe preeclampsia. The relative risks for ischemic heart disease were 1.48, 1.57, 1.61, for heart failure were 1.37, 1.67, 1.71, for stroke were 1.51, 1.43, 1.58, for thromboembolism were 1.03, 1.53, 1.91, and for type 2 diabetes were 3.12, 3.53, 3.68 for gestational hypertension, mild preeclampsia, and severe preeclampsia, respectively. This study demonstrates that preeclampsia is a common risk factor for a multitude of differing medical diagnoses.

The cumulative experience strongly suggests that preeclampsia can be used to predict future vascular disease and death. Bellamy and colleagues performed a systematic review which included a dataset of approximately 3.5 million women with 198 252 women identified with preeclampsia. Following preeclampsia, there was an increased risk of hypertension (RR, 3.70; 95% CI, 2.7–5.05), ischemic heart disease (RR, 2.16; 95% CI, 1.86–2.52), stroke (RR, 1.81; 95% CI, 1.45–2.27), and venous thromboembolism (RR, 1.79; 95% CI, 1.37–2.33). Overall mortality after preeclampsia was increased with a relative risk of 1.49 (95% CI, 1.05–2.14). There was no increased risk of cancer [11].

These findings offer a strong link between preeclampsia and a future risk of CVD and other adverse maternal outcomes. The association is greatest with earlier and more "severe" disease. In summary, the observation of a normal blood pressure after preeclampsia should not discourage the search for other cardiovascular risk factors or abrogate the need for other preventive measures. Multiple episodes of preeclampsia or early-onset preeclampsia should heighten the awareness of primary care physicians even more. These observations may ultimately shed light on the pathogenesis of preeclampsia, and may ultimately identify subgroups of women at highest risk of heart disease, whose risk may be favorably modified by increased screening intervals as well as appropriate preventive measures.

■ The link between preeclampsia and cardiovascular disease: proposed explanations

How preeclampsia results in CVD risk remains a mystery. Clearly, both conditions share many risk factors (discussed in Chapters 2 and 4). Some commonly accepted risk factors for both conditions include: increasing maternal age [12,13], chronic hypertension [14], diabetes [12,15,16], a maternal hypercoaguable state [17–21], and elevated serum homocysteine levels [22]. Common manifestations of the metabolic syndrome have also been related to both preeclampsia and CVD including: androgen excess including polycystic ovarian syndrome [23], elevated testosterone [24], male fat distribution (increased waist-to-hip ratio) [25], dyslipidemia [26], lipoprotein lipase mutations [27], and obesity. In a prospective study, Magnussen *et al.* [28] examined common risk factors for CVD prior to pregnancy in 3494 Norwegian women and demonstrated that women with these risk factors were at increased risk for developing preeclampsia. These risk factors included elevated pre-pregnancy triglycerides, cholesterol, and blood pressure.

Pregnancy as a stress test

Although common risk factors between preeclampsia and CVD are sure to play some role in their close association, others have postulated that pregnancy may be a "stress test" where preeclampsia, similar to gestational diabetes, is a manifestation of previously occult pathology that becomes clinically visible due to the numerous physiological stresses of pregnancy. Similar to any stress test, normal pregnancy involves a dramatic increase in renal function and cardiac output, insulin resistance, hyperlipidemia, thrombotic potential, and the upregulation of inflammation, all of which place a stress on the renal system, various maternal endocrine pathways, and cardiovascular homeostasis. After the pregnancy stress is removed, clinical manifestations of disease remit, but the increased vulnerability remains. This vulnerability, combined with physiological stresses of aging, obesity, development of comorbidities, and other pathology, makes women more likely to develop clinical disorders such as diabetes and CVD.

Endothelial dysfunction

Although the pathogenesis of preeclampsia remains uncertain, endothelial dysfunction clearly plays a prominent role in both preeclampsia and CVD. Systemic dysfunction can explain most of the signs and symptoms of preeclampsia and, in part, may be caused by an imbalance of angiogenic factors such as vascular endothelial growth factor (VEGF) and placental growth factor (PlGF) and anti-angiogenic factors such as sFlt-1 [29].

Most studies have demonstrated persistent endothelial dysfunction with preeclampsia during pregnancy [30,31] or in the postpartum period after preeclampsia. Chambers *et al.* [32] demonstrated, in a case–control study, that women with a history of preeclampsia when compared with women with uncomplicated pregnancies had significant endothelial dysfunction. Cases were a median of 3 years postpartum. Brachial artery flow-mediated, endothelium-dependent dilatation was lower in women with a history of preeclampsia compared with controls. This reduction was even more pronounced in women with recurrent preeclampsia. Similar results have been described by others and would suggest a predisposition to hypertension, atherosclerosis, and ultimately CVD [33–35].

Studies concerning endothelial dysfunction have not yet included an assessment of women prior to becoming pregnant, thereby impairing our understanding of the connection between preeclampsia and CVD. Although it appears clear that endothelial dysfunction is a persistent feature in women with a history of preeclampsia, without data prior to pregnancy, it remains difficult to determine whether endothelial dysfunction is a consequence of preeclampsia that ultimately leads to CVD or alternatively a subclinical process that may exist prior to pregnancy that blossoms into preeclampsia due to the "stress test" of pregnancy and again many years later as CVD.

Metabolic syndrome and insulin resistance

Beyond endothelial dysfunction, preeclampsia is accompanied by multiple features that are common to metabolic syndrome including: hypertension, hyperinsulinemia, glucose intolerance, obesity, lipid abnormalities, increased leptin, increased tumor necrosis factor-alpha (TNFα), increased tissue plasminogen activator antigen (TPA-Ag) and plasminogen activator inhibitor-1 (PAI-1), increased testosterone, and reduced sex hormone-binding globulin [36].

Insulin resistance may have particular importance for preeclampsia as it is associated with the activation of the sympathetic nervous system, modified cation transport, and renal sodium retention [37,38], as well as endothelial dysfunction [39], which may all contribute to hypertension during pregnancy. It is well recognized that normal pregnancy is an insulin-resistant and hyperinsulinemic state that is progressive through gestation and these changes are exaggerated during preeclamptic pregnancy [40,41]. Furthermore, these alterations in insulin physiology persist at a higher rate beyond pregnancy in women with a preeclampsia history and may be another link to CVD [42,43]. Beyond persistent insulin resistance, cholesterol and triglycerides levels also remain higher than in non-preeclamptic women in the postpartum period [44].

Unfortunately, there are few studies that have well-addressed the insulin status prior to pregnancy, making it difficult to determine the primary insult. However, cross-sectional studies allude to a hyperinsulinemic state prior to the onset of clinical disease, though again, these studies may simply be identifying subclinical preeclampsia. Clinically however, we know that insulin-resistant states such as type 2 diabetes, gestational diabetes, and metabolic syndrome prior to pregnancy are risk factors for both preeclampsia and CVD [12]. Due to the similar features of metabolic syndrome and preeclampsia, some hypothesize that preeclampsia may be an early manifestation of the metabolic syndrome in a similar fashion as gestational diabetes is for diabetes in later life. The progressive insulin resistance during pregnancy may be a stress test that predisposes to clinical preeclampsia in women with underlying insulin resistance/metabolic disease [36,45].

Epidemiological studies now support a connection between insulin resistance, preeclampsia, and CVD. Lykke *et al.* demonstrated an association between preeclampsia and future CVD as well as diabetes development in later life and strengthens the argument that underlying insulin resistance may be an integral part of the increased CVD risk [10].

Inflammation

One possible mechanism that could underlie the "stress test" of pregnancy is the inflammatory cascade. A patient's genetically or environmentally determined pro-inflammatory phenotype may be unmasked by the physiological increase in inflammatory response seen in all pregnancies, which may lead to clinically diagnosed preeclampsia. Elevated levels of C-reactive protein (CRP), a marker of underlying systemic inflammation, strongly predict future myocardial infarction, stroke, vascular events [46], insulin resistance [47], and the metabolic syndrome [48]. One study found that first-trimester CRP levels were significantly higher among women who later developed preeclampsia [49]. The elevated CRP levels appear to persist in women who have had eclampsia and could be another factor that helps us understand preeclampsia and its relation to CVD [50]. This same study demonstrated a strong relationship with CRP levels and insulin resistance in postmenopausal women after preeclampsia. In sum, low-grade systemic inflammation, as measured by CRP, appears to be involved in the pathogenesis of insulin resistance and preeclampsia, as well as CVD.

■ Conclusion

Common obstetrical complications such as preeclampsia and gestational diabetes appear to be strong predictors of future disease. There now exists a strong argument for non-obstetricians to include these complications in routine history taking to assess an individual risk for CVD and diabetes and this information should be used to guide the strength of preventive health recommendations. Unfortunately, the mechanism of the association remains unclear and whether preeclampsia is merely an expression of subclinical pathology or the cause of permanent injury that results in CVD remains to be delineated.

REFERENCES

1. Barker DJ. Fetal origins of coronary heart disease. *BMJ* 1995;**311**(6998):171–4.

2. Sattar N, Greer IA. Pregnancy complications and maternal cardiovascular risk: opportunities for intervention and screening? *BMJ* 2002;**325**(7356):157–60.

3. Gifford R, August PA, Cunningham G, *et al. The National High Blood Pressure Education Program Working Group on High Blood Pressure in Pregnancy.* Bethesda, National Institutes of Health and National Heart, Lung and Blood Institute, 2000.

4. Chesley SC, Annitto JE, Cosgrove RA. The remote prognosis of eclamptic women. Sixth periodic report. *Am J Obstet Gynecol* 1976;**124**(5):446–59.

5. Sibai BM, el-Nazer A, Gonzalez-Ruiz A. Severe preeclampsia-eclampsia in young primigravid women: subsequent pregnancy outcome and remote prognosis. *Am J Obstet Gynecol* 1986;**155**(5):1011–16.

6. Irgens HU, Reisaeter L, Irgens LM, Lie RT. Long term mortality of mothers and fathers after pre-eclampsia: population based cohort study. *BMJ* 2001; **323**(7323):1213–17.

7. Smith GC, Pell JP, Walsh D. Pregnancy complications and maternal risk of ischaemic heart disease: a retrospective cohort study of 129,290 births. *Lancet* 2001;**357**(9273):2002–6.

8. Funai EF, Friedlander Y, Paltiel O, *et al.* Long-term mortality after preeclampsia. *Epidemiology* 2005;**16**(2):206–15.

9. Vikse BE, Irgens LM, Leivestad T, Skjaerven R, Iversen BM. Preeclampsia and the risk of end-stage renal disease. *N Engl J Med* 2008;**359**(8):800–9.

10. Lykke JA, Langhoff-Roos J, Sibai BM, *et al.* Hypertensive pregnancy disorders and subsequent cardiovascular morbidity and type 2 diabetes mellitus in the mother. *Hypertension* 2009;**53**(6):944–51.

11. Bellamy L, Casas JP, Hingorani AD, Williams DJ. Pre-eclampsia and risk of cardiovascular disease and cancer in later life: systematic review and meta-analysis. *BMJ* 2007;**335**(7627):974.

12. Duckitt K, Harrington D. Risk factors for pre-eclampsia at antenatal booking: systematic review of controlled studies. *BMJ* 2005;**330**(7491):565.

13. Funai EF, Paltiel OB, Malaspina D, *et al.* Risk factors for pre-eclampsia in nulliparous and parous women: the Jerusalem perinatal study. *Paediatr Perinat Epidemiol* 2005;**19**(1):59–68.

14. Sibai BM, Lindheimer M, Hauth J, *et al.* Risk factors for preeclampsia, abruptio placentae, and adverse neonatal outcomes among women with chronic hypertension. National Institute of Child Health and Human Development Network of Maternal-Fetal Medicine Units. *N Engl J Med* 1998;**339**(10):667–71.

15. Ness RB, Markovic N, Bass D, Harger G, Roberts JM. Family history of hypertension, heart disease, and stroke among women who develop hypertension in pregnancy. *Obstet Gynecol* 2003;**102**(6):1366–71.

16. Qiu C, Williams MA, Leisenring WM, *et al.* Family history of hypertension and type 2 diabetes in relation to preeclampsia risk. *Hypertension* 2003;**41**(3):408–13.

17. Kupferminc MJ, Eldor A, Steinman N, *et al*. Increased frequency of genetic thrombophilia in women with complications of pregnancy. *N Engl J Med* 1999;**340**(1):9–13.

18. Rosendaal FR, Siscovick DS, Schwartz SM, *et al*. A common prothrombin variant (20210 G to A) increases the risk of myocardial infarction in young women. *Blood* 1997;**90**(5):1747–50.

19. Rodie VA, Freeman DJ, Sattar N, Greer IA. Pre-eclampsia and cardiovascular disease: metabolic syndrome of pregnancy? *Atherosclerosis* 2004;**175**(2):189–202.

20. Walker ID. Prothrombotic genotypes and pre-eclampsia. *Thromb Haemost* 2002;**87**(5):777–8.

21. Rosendaal FR, Siscovick DS, Schwartz SM, *et al*. Factor V Leiden (resistance to activated protein C) increases the risk of myocardial infarction in young women. *Blood* 1997;**89**(8):2817–21.

22. Powers RW, Evans RW, Majors AK, *et al*. Plasma homocysteine concentration is increased in preeclampsia and is associated with evidence of endothelial activation. *Am J Obstet Gynecol* 1998;**179**(6 Pt 1):1605–11.

23. Fridstrom M, Nisell H, Sjoblom P, Hillensjo T. Are women with polycystic ovary syndrome at an increased risk of pregnancy-induced hypertension and/or preeclampsia? *Hypertens Pregnancy* 1999;**18**(1):73–80.

24. Acromite MT, Mantzoros CS, Leach RE, Hurwitz J, Dorey LG. Androgens in preeclampsia. *Am J Obstet Gynecol* 1999;**180**(1 Pt 1):60–3.

25. Sattar N, Clark P, Holmes A, *et al*. Antenatal waist circumference and hypertension risk. *Obstet Gynecol* 2001;**97**(2):268–71.

26. van den Elzen HJ, Wladimiroff JW, Cohen-Overbeek TE, de Bruin AJ, Grobbee DE. Serum lipids in early pregnancy and risk of pre-eclampsia. *Br J Obstet Gynaecol* 1996;**103**(2):117–22.

27. Hubel CA, Roberts JM, Ferrell RE. Association of pre-eclampsia with common coding sequence variations in the lipoprotein lipase gene. *Clin Genet* 1999; **56**(4):289–96.

28. Magnussen EB, Vatten LJ, Lund-Nilsen TI, *et al*. Prepregnancy cardiovascular risk factors as predictors of pre-eclampsia: population based cohort study. *BMJ* 2007;**335**(7627):978.

29. Widmer M, Villar J, Benigni A, *et al*. Mapping the theories of preeclampsia and the role of angiogenic factors: a systematic review. *Obstet Gynecol* 2007; **109**(1):168–80.

30. Cockell AP, Poston L. Flow-mediated vasodilatation is enhanced in normal pregnancy but reduced in preeclampsia. *Hypertension* 1997;**30**(2 Pt 1):247–51.

31. Savvidou MD, Hingorani AD, Tsikas D, *et al*. Endothelial dysfunction and raised plasma concentrations of asymmetric dimethylarginine in pregnant women who subsequently develop pre-eclampsia. *Lancet* 2003;**361**(9368):1511–17.

32. Chambers JC, Fusi L, Malik IS, *et al*. Association of maternal endothelial dysfunction with preeclampsia. *JAMA* 2001;**285**(12):1607–12.

33. Agatisa PK, Ness RB, Roberts JM, *et al*. Impairment of endothelial function in women with a history of preeclampsia: an indicator of cardiovascular risk. *Am J Physiol Heart Circ Physiol* 2004;**286**(4):H1389–93.

34. Spaanderman ME, Willekes C, Hoeks AP, Ekhart TH, Peeters LL. The effect of pregnancy on the compliance of large arteries and veins in healthy parous control subjects and women with a history of preeclampsia. *Am J Obstet Gynecol* 2000;**183**(5):1278–86.

35. Lampinen KH, Ronnback M, Kaaja RJ, Groop PH. Impaired vascular dilatation in women with a history of pre-eclampsia. *J Hypertens* 2006;**24**(4):751–6.

36. Seely EW, Solomon CG. Insulin resistance and its potential role in pregnancy-induced hypertension. *J Clin Endocrinol Metab* 2003;**88**(6):2393–8.

37. Solomon CG, Seely EW. Brief review: hypertension in pregnancy: a manifestation of the insulin resistance syndrome? *Hypertension* 2001;**37**(2):232–9.

38. Reaven GM. Pathophysiology of insulin resistance in human disease. *Physiol Rev* 1995;**75**(3):473–86.

39. Wheatcroft SB, Williams IL, Shah AM, Kearney MT. Pathophysiological implications of insulin resistance on vascular endothelial function. *Diabet Med* 2003;**20**(4):255–68.

40. Butte NF. Carbohydrate and lipid metabolism in pregnancy: normal compared with gestational diabetes mellitus. *Am J Clin Nutr* 2000;**71**(5 Suppl):1256S–61S.

41. Kaaja R, Tikkanen MJ, Viinikka L, Ylikorkala O. Serum lipoproteins, insulin, and urinary prostanoid metabolites in normal and hypertensive pregnant women. *Obstet Gynecol* 1995;**85**(3):353–6.

42. Laivuori H, Tikkanen MJ, Ylikorkala O. Hyperinsulinemia 17 years after preeclamptic first pregnancy. *J Clin Endocrinol Metab* 1996;**81**(8):2908–11.

43. Wolf M, Hubel CA, Lam C, *et al.* Preeclampsia and future cardiovascular disease: potential role of altered angiogenesis and insulin resistance. *J Clin Endocrinol Metab* 2004;**89**(12):6239–43.

44. Smith GN, Walker MC, Liu A, *et al.* A history of preeclampsia identifies women who have underlying cardiovascular risk factors. *Am J Obstet Gynecol* 2009;**200**(1):58.e1–8.

45. Kaaja RJ, Greer IA. Manifestations of chronic disease during pregnancy. *JAMA* 2005;**294**(21):2751–7.

46. Willerson JT, Ridker PM. Inflammation as a cardiovascular risk factor. *Circulation* 2004;**109**(21 Suppl 1):II2–10.

47. Sjoholm A, Nystrom T. Endothelial inflammation in insulin resistance. *Lancet* 2005;**365**(9459):610–12.

48. Ridker PM, Buring JE, Cook NR, Rifai N. C-reactive protein, the metabolic syndrome, and risk of incident cardiovascular events: an 8-year follow-up of 14 719 initially healthy American women. *Circulation* 2003;**107**(3):391–7.

49. Vickers M, Ford I, Morrison R, *et al.* Markers of endothelial activation and atherothrombosis in women with history of preeclampsia or gestational hypertension. *Thromb Haemost* 2003;**90**(6):1192–7.

50. Hubel CA, Powers RW, Snaedal S, *et al.* C-reactive protein is elevated 30 years after eclamptic pregnancy. *Hypertension* 2008;**51**(6):1499–505.

Index